CRANIAL
OSTEOPATHIC BIOMECHANICS, PATHOMECHANICS AND DIAGNOSTICS FOR PRACTITIONERS

Dedication

To my patients
who by entrusting themselves to my hands have allowed me to learn; who by improving have allowed me to understand; who by being cured allow me to pass on the lesson they have taught me. Therapy is the art of uniting and separating, the result of a shared act.

Senior Commissioning Editor: Sarena Wolfaard
Associate Editor: Claire Wilson
Project Manager: Jess Thompson
Design Direction: Stewart Larking
Illustrator: René Lavatelli

CRANIAL
OSTEOPATHIC BIOMECHANICS, PATHOMECHANICS AND DIAGNOSTICS FOR PRACTITIONERS

by *Alain Géhin*

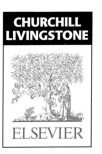

CHURCHILL LIVINGSTONE

ELSEVIER

Edinburgh London New York Oxford Philadelphia St Louis Sydney Toronto 2007

CHURCHILL
LIVINGSTONE
ELSEVIER

An imprint of Elsevier Limited

© Masson, Paris 2005
© 2007, Elsevier Limited. All rights reserved.

The right of Alain Géhin to be identified as author of this work has been asserted by him in accordance with the Copyright, Designs and Patents Act 1988.

First edition 2005 (French edition)
First edition 2007

ISBN: 978-0-08-045114-5

British Library Cataloguing in Publication Data
A catalogue record for this book is available from the British Library

Library of Congress Cataloging in Publication Data
A catalog record for this book is available from the Library of Congress

Note
Neither the Publisher nor the Author assume any responsibility for any loss or injury and/or damage to persons or property arising out of or related to any use of the material contained in this book. It is the responsibility of the treating practitioner, relying on independent expertise and knowledge of the patient, to determine the best treatment and method of application for the patient.

The Publisher

Printed in China

Contents

While respecting anatomy as closely as possible, the diagrams throughout the book reflect an anatomical ideal and make no claim whatsoever to replace or supplant courses in anatomy or physiology.

• *Figure 1*

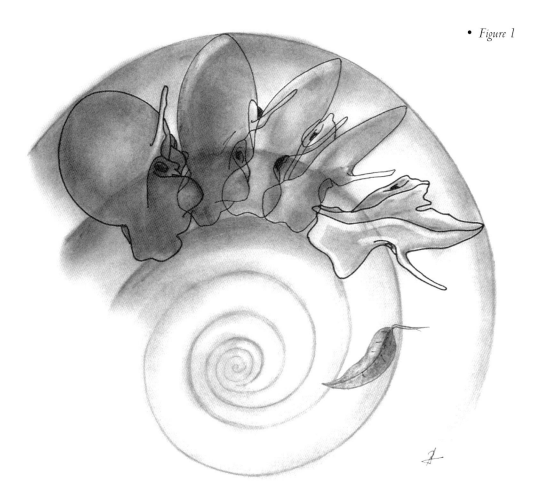

The cardioid is the geometrical figure that represents the locus of the different axes of a movement in space: it is the essence of movement.

Introduction

Any medical approach to health problems by manual treatment must have a very firm basis, which is provided here by cranial anatomy and biomechanics. There is certainly a wealth of reliable literature on anatomy, but unfortunately biomechanics is less well documented: the references are sporadic, incomplete, and sparse in the few publications devoted to this discipline. So there is really no overview that would allow the detailed research that would be so useful in this field.

This lack is perhaps due to the fact that numerous approaches to cranial technique are based on the development of perception during the teaching period. Although this is undeniably necessary in order to acquire manual ability, it seems inadequate to understand pathomechanics, which must form the basis of the reasoning that leads practitioners to the choice of techniques they intend to use.

In fact, how is it possible to understand pathomechanics without having a previous knowledge of biomechanics?

We have therefore assembled in this book all that we have found useful in thirty years of teaching cranial technique in ten countries. The contents seem to us to be the basic minimum necessary to understand cranial biomechanics.

It is already more than ten years since the publication of our first book on cranial manipulation; since then, it has been translated into ten languages. We delayed the planned publication of the second book because cranial technique, even in the most expert hands, seemed to us insufficient for dealing with all basically reversible lesions that could be treated efficiently.

The last ten years have given us the opportunity to find technical manual solutions to the rising tide of traumas, many of which are caused by the mechanical civilization in which we live.

Over these ten years, we have been able, through experience shared with our many patients, to refine very precisely the biomechanics that our predecessors introduced to us and guided us through.

Also over these ten years, we have come to realize that the general techniques used previously were sometimes not precise enough, and that specific techniques were not always perfectly adapted to the general body of knowledge. This led us to perfect other better adapted techniques, especially when several joints were involved. Such techniques had not been used previously, but they allowed progression from the particular to the general without altering either the specificity or the totality of a method that takes into account the wholeness of a human being.

To improve its usefulness, we describe in this work manual exploratory techniques that can uncover functional defects of the cranial system and their pathomechanical characteristics. And this allows the practitioner to choose the most suitable techniques through reference to our book *Atlas of Techniques of Manipulation for the Bones of the Skull and Face.*

In this book, we have laid out the basic techniques that we have devised, improved, and developed during thirty years of practice. This long period of gradual development through practice will soon result in a complete revision of this book in order to include the results of our recent research.

Therefore, a third book will follow, which will give us the opportunity to choose corrective manual techniques that are related to manual perception. Their existing anatomical and physiological bases, together with our knowledge of pathomechanics, will then allow us to understand dysfunctions and their pathological implications.

For the present, however, let us examine the foundations of a manual diagnosis that is simple, clear, and precise in the sensitive hands of trained therapists.

It has been our guiding principle to go from the simple to the complex, leaving each professional to find his own starting point on this road.

Our hope is to help all practitioners who have found their own way of applying cranial osteopathic technique in the manual treatment of their patients' dysfunctions.

General
Points

Anatomy and biomechanics

Learning the technical aspects of cranial osteopathy is grounded in *anatomy*, which constitutes its structural substrate, and in *biomechanics*, which provides its functional component.

Mastery of these techniques will then follow as a result of progressive refinement of one's proprioception, as regards both the plasticity of the bones and the mini-movements that take place at the sutures.

As for all senses, proprioception begins at the level of a sensor that transmits information to the primary centers of the brain and then on to the secondary centers, which refine its interpretation according to predetermined tactile systems of reference.

Therefore, learning will consist of a constant expansion of these systems of reference thanks to continuous exposure to tactile sensations and to the attention devoted to them, i.e., the reinforcement process of training.

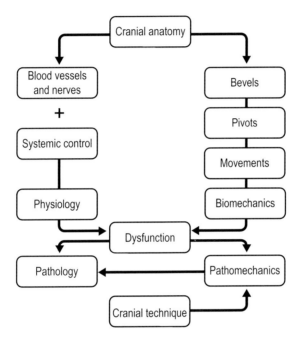

The arterial blood supply

Everyone knows that the brain has a high rate of consumption of blood-borne oxygen and glucose. We need only look at the internal aspect of a bone of the cranial vault to observe how extensively it is grooved by the imprints of blood vessels.

As shown by Professor Lazorthe, the arterial supply to the brain has specific and distinctive characteristics. Thus, unlike many organs, the brain has numerous arterial pedicles because its arterial blood supply comes from four large vessels (i.e., two carotid arteries and two vertebral arteries).

These arteries anastomose to form the arterial circle of Willis, from which arise the cerebral arteries. The cerebral arteries then give rise to two systems of blood supply to the brain:

- the first, made up of the cortical branches, coats the external surface of the brain;
- the second, consisting of the central branches, enters the brain at its core.

These two systems of arterial branches then penetrate the brain substance, with the vessels of one system running towards the point of entry of the vessels of the other system and thinning progressively along their course. Hence, the two most vascular zones of the cerebrum are cortical and central.

These vessels branch further in the brain substance, with each branch supplying a well-defined territory. As Professor Lazorthe puts it, "The distribution of the cerebral arteries to separate anastomotic territories suggests the existence of juxtaposed but cofunctional hemodynamic currents." In addition, there is no mixing of the blood carried by the anterior, middle, and posterior cerebral arteries where they join the circle of Willis, and their supply to the brain is strictly ipsilateral.

It may be useful to recall that each lateral surface of the body of the sphenoid contains a sulcus for the internal carotid artery as it traverses the cavernous sinus, to which it is attached by fibrous bands.

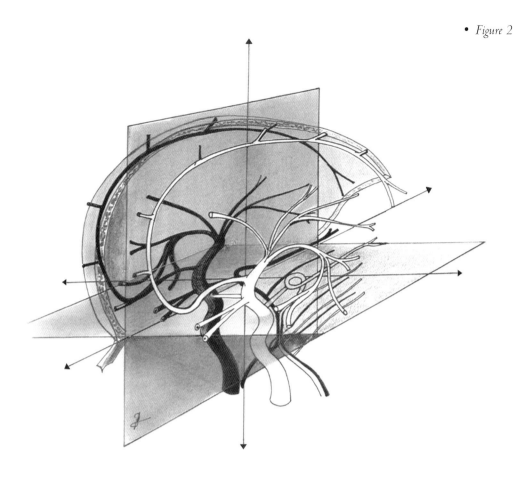

• *Figure 2*

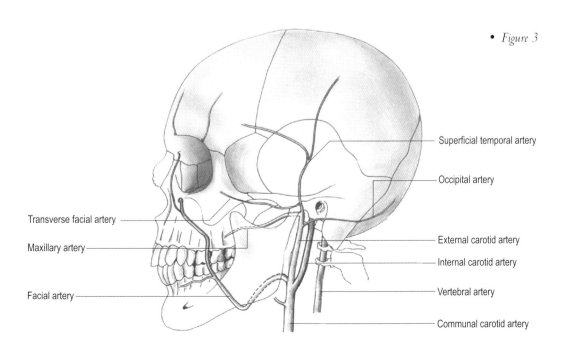

• *Figure 3*

Superficial temporal artery

Occipital artery

Transverse facial artery

Maxillary artery

Facial artery

External carotid artery

Internal carotid artery

Vertebral artery

Communal carotid artery

We believe that the possible effects of each of our cranial techniques can be explained by the presence of vascular grooves in the cranial bones and by the intracranial organization of the arteries, including the formation of the circle of Willis at the base of the brain, the peripheral disposition of the vessels, the highly segmental blood supply to the brain, and the attachment of the internal carotid to the body of the sphenoid.

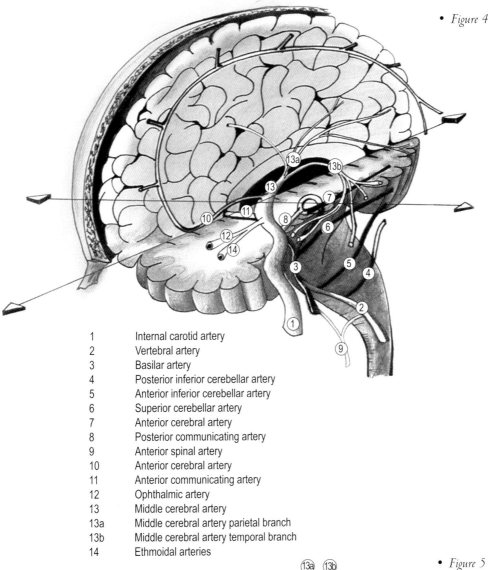

• *Figure 4*

1	Internal carotid artery
2	Vertebral artery
3	Basilar artery
4	Posterior inferior cerebellar artery
5	Anterior inferior cerebellar artery
6	Superior cerebellar artery
7	Anterior cerebral artery
8	Posterior communicating artery
9	Anterior spinal artery
10	Anterior cerebral artery
11	Anterior communicating artery
12	Ophthalmic artery
13	Middle cerebral artery
13a	Middle cerebral artery parietal branch
13b	Middle cerebral artery temporal branch
14	Ethmoidal arteries

• *Figure 5*

Main branches of the internal carotid and vertebral arteries

Diagrams based on *Anatomie Humaine* by J.-W. Rohen, C. Yokochi Vigot, 2nd edition

Distribution of the cranial and cerebral arteries

Examination of the grooves made on the endocranium by the *meningeal vessels* reveals a fan-like arrangement, facing posteriorly, which developed during phylogenesis in conjunction with rotation of the occiput.

Likewise, the distribution of the cerebral arteries in the different areas of the brain exhibits a very distinctive topography.

Radiographic studies of the *cerebral arteries*, which are commonly carried out nowadays, indicate that all the arterial branches run posteriorly as if swept along by a gust of wind.

All these vessels arise from the circle of Willis plastered against the cranial base. After ascending for a short distance, they all curve backwards to run posteriorly.

The same applies to the *middle cerebral artery*. The *anterior cerebral arteries* ascend for a short distance toward the frontal lobe before turning backward.

The venous circulation

Generally speaking, the venous circulation runs alongside the arteries at certain key points (i.e., the intracavernous portion of the internal carotid, the intracerebral arteries, etc.). Furthermore, some venous sinuses enjoy a special relationship with the cranial vault: the *superior sagittal sinus* lying at the site of insertion of the falx cerebri into the lips of the sagittal suture, the *straight sinus* similarly inserted into the squamous part of the occipital bone, the confluence of sinuses related to the lambdoid suture, etc.

As these veins have no valves, we think that the venous return is influenced by movements at the sutures and also by the plasticity of the lamellar or *squamous* bones, particularly in the cranial vault.

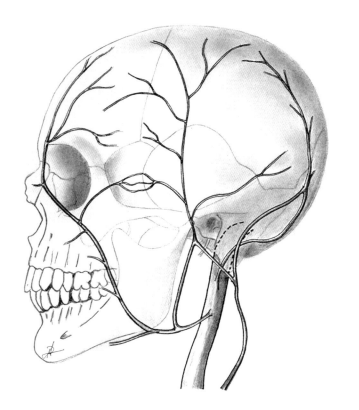

• *Figure 6*

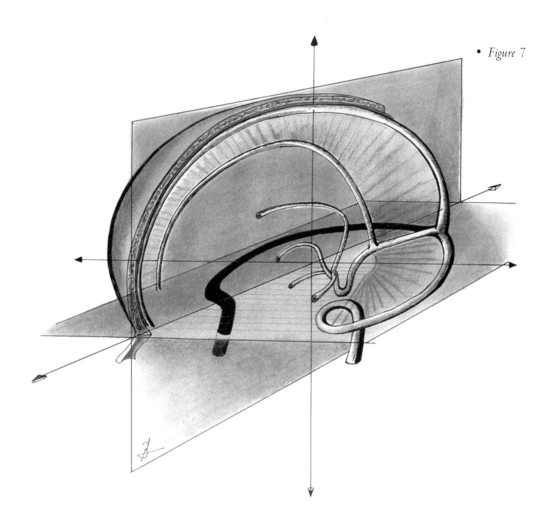

• *Figure* 7

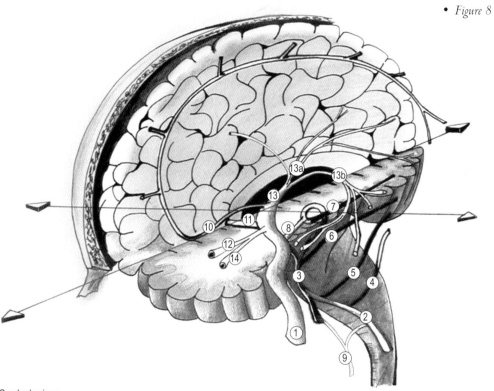

• *Figure 8*

Cerebral veins :
1. Superior longitudinal sinus
2. Inferior longitudinal sinus
3. Straight sinus
4. Great cerebral vein (great cerebral vein of Galen)
5. Internal cerebral veins
6. Basal veins
7. Lateral sinuses

Section through the cranial base (with the sutures opened)

This section with the sutures opened shows right away that the central position is occupied by the spheno-basilar (spheno-occipital) synchondrosis lying between the anterior part of the occipital bone and the posterior part of the body of the sphenoid.

Professor Tamboise (Paris, 1985) has identified the presence of differentiated cells in the adult spheno-basilar synchondrosis that respond to various forces as a result of their elasticity. Its plasticity, reinforced by the plasticity of the other sutures, provides enough support for the osteopaths' belief in the dynamic nature of the cranium.

It is amusing to note that the two bones forming this synchondrosis bear two different names, despite opponents of this dynamic notion of the cranium referring to the development of a physiological synostosis at around 25 years of age. Would there be two names for the same bone?

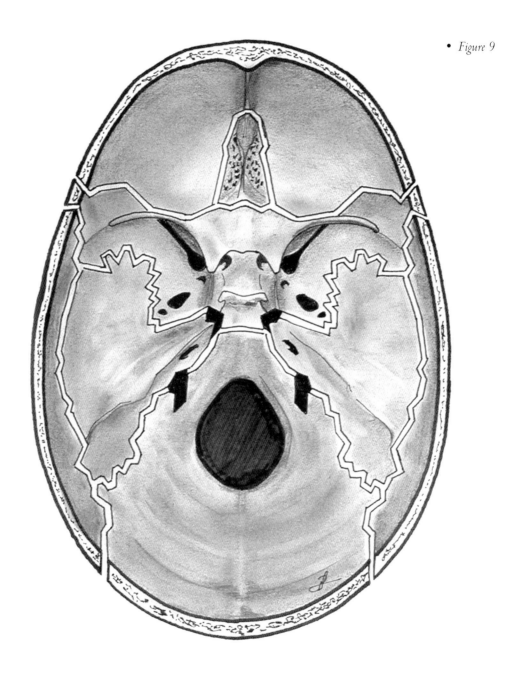

• *Figure 9*

Lateral view of the cranium (with the sutures opened)

This lateral view of the cranium with the sutures opened clearly shows the following:

- the general pattern of the sutures as well as their location;
- the spatial location of the spheno-basilar synchondrosis;
- the triangular shape of the temporal bone, with its base lying laterally and its apex flanking the two bones of this synchondrosis;
- the lateral line of force that runs from the mastoid through the zygomatic process to reach the zygomatic bone and the maxilla.

It is worth stressing that this tight triangular articulation, which unites these two bones, is intensely denticulate.

In order to complete our description of the cranial system and, in particular, to illustrate the location of each of its constituent bones, we include two three-quarter views of the skull, the first (Fig. 11) unaltered and the second (Fig. 12) expanded with the sutures opened.

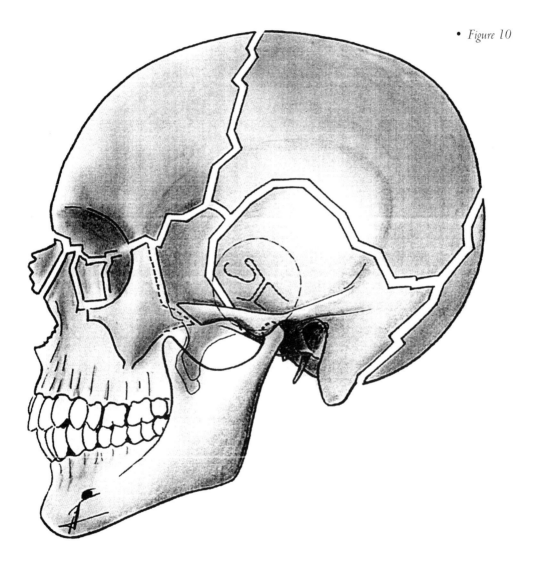

• *Figure 10*

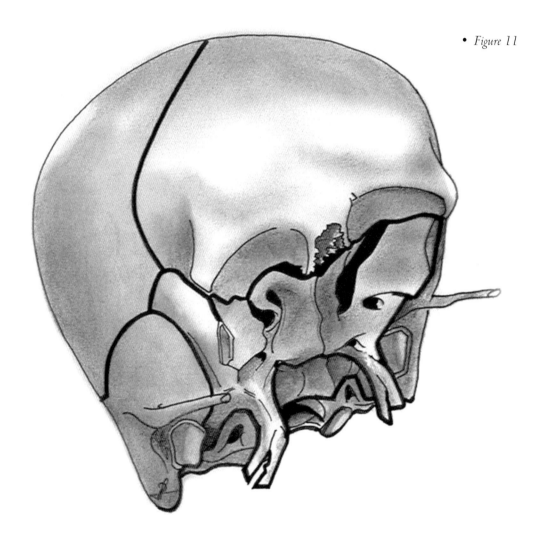

• *Figure 11*

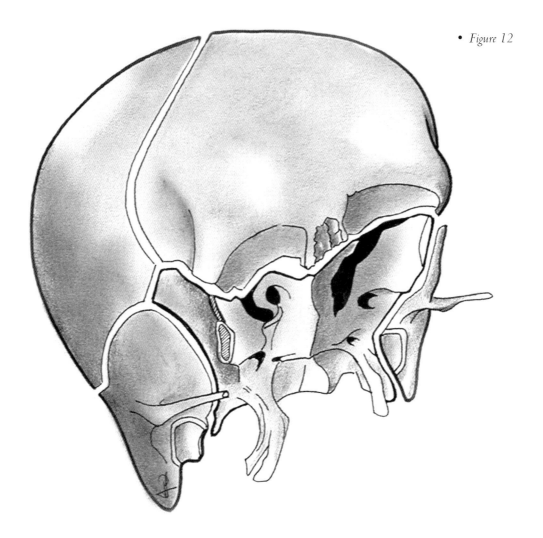

• *Figure 12*

The embryological basis

The cranium is made up of two different embryological primordia:

- the first, of membranous origin, forms the *vault*, which is the most malleable part;
- the second, of cartilaginous origin, is more solid and forms the base.

On the inner surface of the junction of these components, the *tentorium cerebelli* is inserted, which, along with the *falx cerebri*, forms the so-called reciprocal tension membranes; these membranes act to balance out the dynamic distortions that arise rhythmically as a result of the movements of the cranial bones.

These three distinct structures carry lines of force that ensure that shocks are propagated and dissipated into the denser cranial bones, e.g., the maxilla, the mastoids, etc.

We know that cranial dynamics must be viewed as an *evolving process* because they are slightly altered in accordance with the progressive ossification of the various components of the cranium, particularly of the sutures.

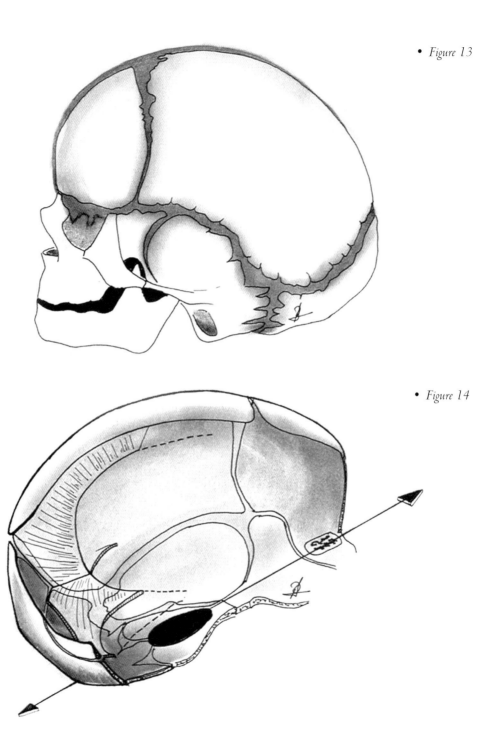

• *Figure 13*

• *Figure 14*

PART ONE

Cranial
Biomechanics

Basic principles

The whole field of articular biomechanics is based on three systems that act concomitantly and synchronously:

- an **intra-articular passive dynamic system** that allows and limits movement and distributes forces in response to the balancing system;
- a **balancing system** that regulates and harmonizes the actions already mentioned;
- an **extra-articular active dynamic system** that induces movement.

Of course, our diagnostic and therapeutic manipulation will act only on the first two systems. We will therefore study *cranial articulation* first, followed by the *balancing system.*

Anatomy of cranial articulation

As shown on the opposite page, cranial articulation consists of the same components that are present in every other joint in the human body. These components are set in motion by internal and external forces, which are constantly balanced by internal forces.

Cranial articulation consists of the following:

- **sliding surfaces** (beveled and squamous sutures), either separate (denticulate sutures) or juxtaposed (harmonic sutures);
- **an overlying periosteum**;
- **restoring ligaments**, formed by the bifurcation of the insertions of the tentorium cerebelli and the falx cerebri and their attachments on either side of a suture;
- **a free nerve ending** in the sutural space, as demonstrated in 1992 by a study performed in the Anatomy Department of the University of Michigan (*Nerve fibres and endings in cranial sutures*, Ernest W. Retzglaff, Fred L. Mitchell Jr., John E. Upledger, and Thomas Biggert);
- **intrasutural arteries and veins**;
- **intrasutural proprioceptors** (Bunt, South Africa, 1996).

It is unlikely that a part of the body so well equipped with typical articular components is intended to remain fixed.

Indeed, it is even more unlikely given that Professor Tamboise showed in 1985 that the sutures contained many osteoblasts, reflecting their constant activity.

This demonstrates the existence of cranial articulation and its dynamic nature. It justifies *per se* our predecessors' concept of cranial osteopathy, even if modern techniques developed since their time were solely responsible for establishing its scientific basis, and the PhD thesis in medical engineering by our colleague Jean-Claude Herriou (*The sutures and mechanical properties of the cranial bones*) has provided valuable scientific proof.

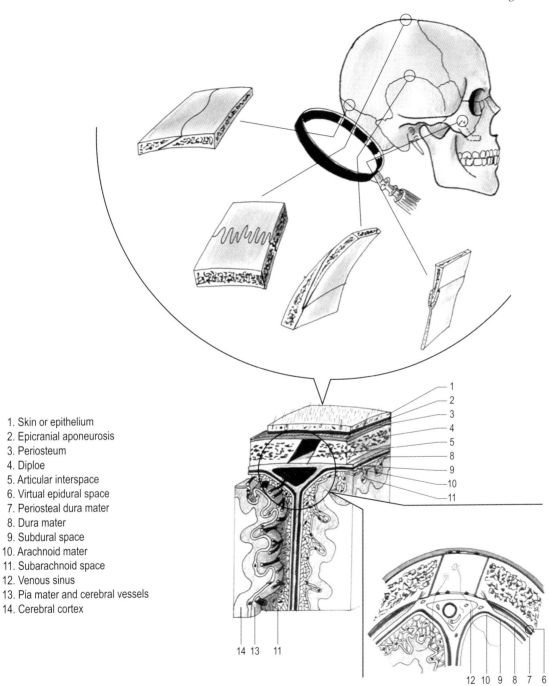

• *Figure 15*

1. Skin or epithelium
2. Epicranial aponeurosis
3. Periosteum
4. Diploe
5. Articular interspace
6. Virtual epidural space
7. Periosteal dura mater
8. Dura mater
9. Subdural space
10. Arachnoid mater
11. Subarachnoid space
12. Venous sinus
13. Pia mater and cerebral vessels
14. Cerebral cortex

29

The three cranial subsystems

As a result of their different embryological origins, their variable resistance to the lines of force, and their variable involvement in cranial dynamics, there are three biodynamic subsystems:

- the **cranial base**, of cartilaginous origin, is strong and resistant and is considered to be the *motor* component;
- the **cranial vault**, of membranous origin, is more flexible and clearly more malleable and is considered to be the *adaptive component*;
- the **face** is not unified by bones of membranous origin and is more mobile; it is the *expressive component*.

The motor cranial base

This is of cartilaginous origin, is viewed as the generator of cranial motion, and is located at the spheno-basilar synchondrosis (i.e., between the posterior part of the body of the sphenoid and the anterior part of the basilar portion of the occipital bone).

The lines of force that run through its bony constituents are multidirectional and consist of longitudinal and transverse beams, as well as buttresses that ensure the dynamic plasticity of the cranial base.

Its resistance is due to the density of its composite pillars and beams.

According to Beryl E. Arbuckle, the lines of force (also called the lines of stress) embedded in the dura mater are continuous with those in the bones.

Attached to the cranial base are the spinal and cranial membranes and the fascial sheets of the neck, which are continuous throughout the body as a unified structure.

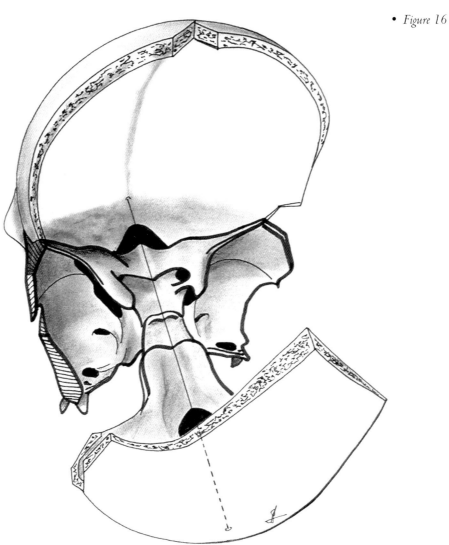

• *Figure 16*

The adaptable vault

As a result of its membranous origin, the cranial vault, with its many sutures, is the major adapter mechanically.

The flexibility of the vault is due to the lamellar shape of its constituent bones or bone fragments and to its heterogeneous components being resistant to creeping and bending movements.

Moreover, the internal membranes, which balance the movements of the cranial system from birth and, to a progressively lesser degree, throughout life, have lines of force that are anchored to and continuous with those of the cranial base.

The vault is therefore the ultimate dissipator of the effects of all vertical shocks and is able to offset many of the ascending forces that have not already been absorbed. This is the focal point of all vertical anti-gravity forces.

• *Figure 17*

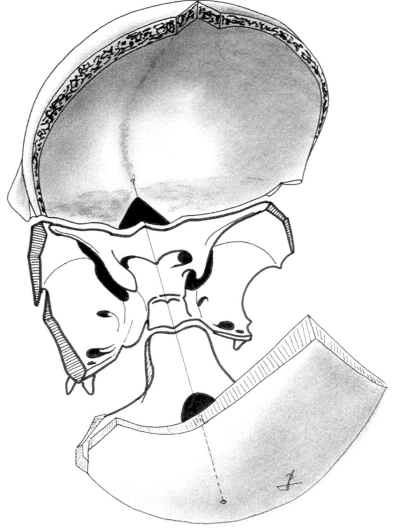

The expressive face

Biomechanically speaking, facial movements are due to the sphenoid and, to a lesser degree, to the temporal bones, and the movements progress via the zygomatic process along the buttress-like lines of force that originate from the mastoid processes.

We know that the facial bones are hung from the frontal bone, which lies in the median plane and participates in movements of flexion–extension.

In the face, the articulations between the various bones are either juxtaposed or serrated but they are not beveled, permitting very localized restriction of movement without necessarily modifying the general pattern of mobility.

Only a change in the central axis (made up of the maxillae, the palatine bones, and the vomer) will have a more widespread effect on mobility, as it articulates with all of the other facial bones. A rich and diverse musculature coupled with multiple articulations is responsible for the wealth and fluidity of facial expressions. Loss of facial expression due to traumatic immobility of the sphenoid is a perfect example of this loss of movement.

• *Figure 18*

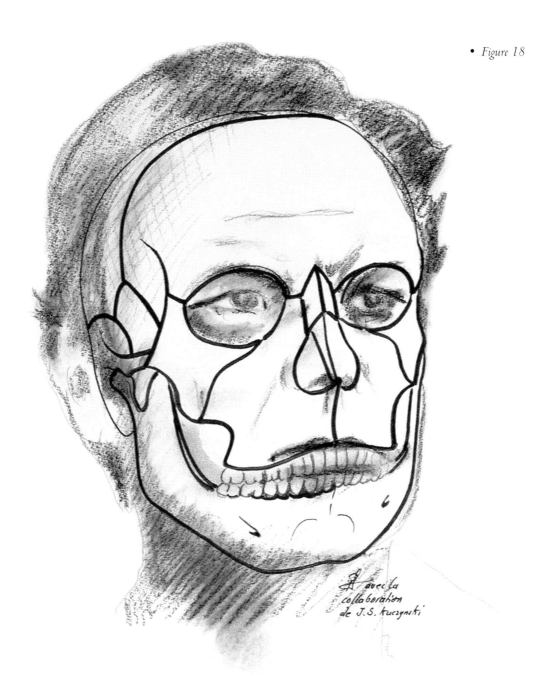

avec la
collaboration
de J.S. Kuczynski

Cranial biomechanics

The biomechanics of cranial mobility

As we have already seen, sutures allow movements between the bones around the axes sited at their pivotal points, which lie where the sutural bevels change orientation.

All cranial bones can be moved by tiny amounts, which combine with the plasticity of the bones to ensure cranial mobility.
These movements take place around three axes: *transverse*, *vertical*, and *antero-posterior*.

Although its curved structure and its sutures allow spatial movement around the three axes, the cranial system mainly shows movement of *flexion–extension* at the level of the centrally located bones (the occipital, sphenoid, frontal, and ethmoid bones and the vomer). These movements occur synchronously with those of the peripheral bones (temporal, parietal, maxillary, and palatine bones and the zygomas) around oblique axes that are specific for each bone and are defined in terms of *external* and *internal rotation*.

The general mobility of the cranial system consists of a cyclical movement with two successive phases:

- an **active phase** combining flexion of the central bones with external rotation of the peripheral bones, called *expansion*;
- a **passive phase** combining extension of the central bones with internal rotation of the peripheral bones, called *relaxation.*

Within this cranial system, each bone will perform a specific movement depending on its axes in the three spatial planes.

Movements of the midline bones

Movements of these bones (unpaired bones and those of the cranial base) take place around three axes – transverse, antero-posterior, and vertical – but preferentially around the transverse axis for each bone.

The movements between these central bones follow those typically seen in a gear system.

The other axes allow a requisite degree of adaptation, which will be discussed later in its commonest manifestations.

• *Figure 19*

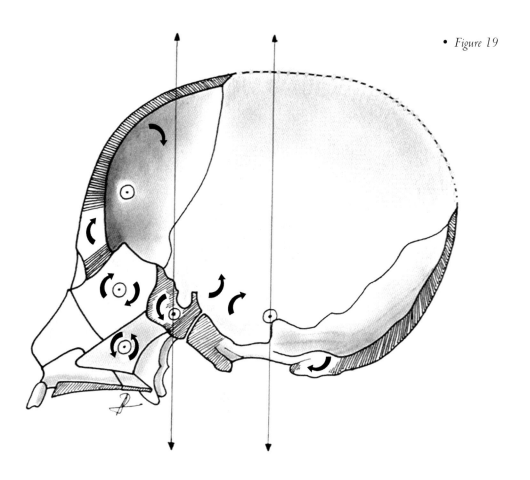

Movements of the occipital bone

The main movement of the occipital bone is that of *flexion–extension* around a transverse axis lying at the intersection of two planes, which pass through the anterior border of the foramen magnum and through the superior border of the basilar portion of the occipital bone. During movement, the part of the bone anterior to this axis is elevated, while its posterior part is displaced inferiorly and anteriorly.

Nonetheless, as we shall make clear with respect to each bone, the occipital bone can also move around its antero-posterior and vertical axes; these movements allow certain functional adaptations to occur.

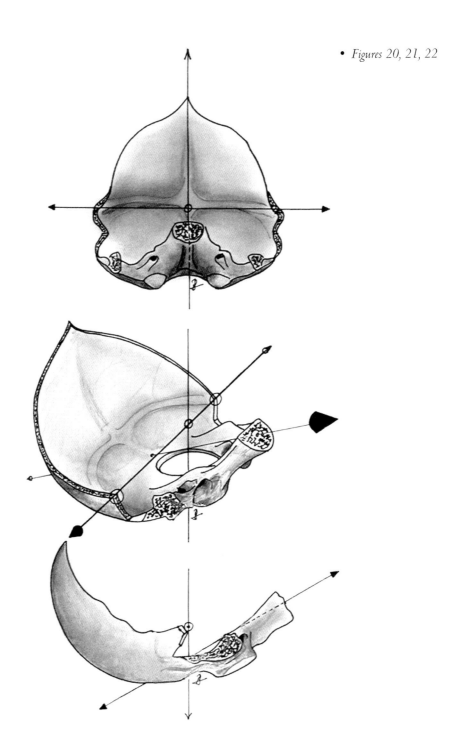

• *Figures 20, 21, 22*

Movements of the sphenoid

The main movement of the sphenoid occurs about its transverse axis in two successive stages:

- first, its body and its greater wings are displaced inferiorly and anteriorly with respect to its main axis, which is located in the middle of its body;
- once this movement has taken place, the greater wings continue to move inferiorly and anteriorly, but this time about a transverse axis running through their roots or sites of attachment to the body.

This second stage thus corresponds to a movement of torsion of the greater wings around their sites of attachment to the body.

Because of its special location at mid-level in the cranium, the sphenoid is often called upon to balance the adaptive movements of the other bones of the cranial base relative to one another by undergoing compensatory movements about its antero-posterior and vertical axes.

Likewise, the plasticity of the roots of the greater wings allows them to adapt their movements to those of the body in different planes.

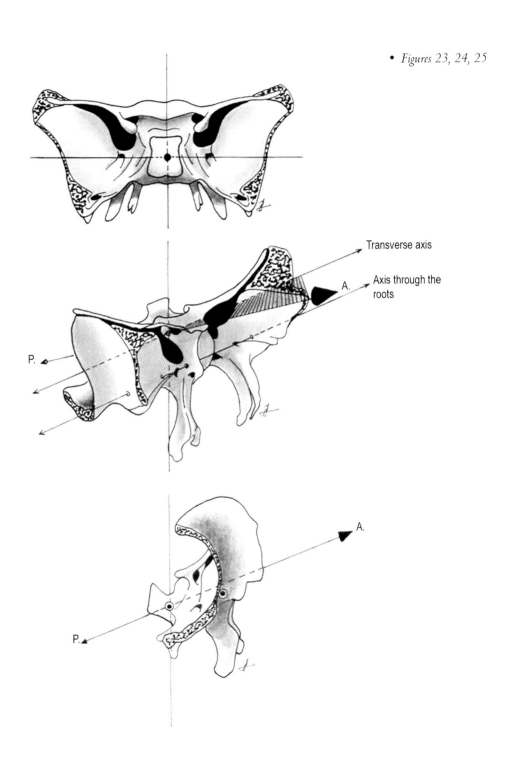

Transverse axis

Axis through the roots

A.

P.

A.

P.

Movement of the spheno-basilar synchondrosis

This joint is deemed to be the underlying motor and starting point of cranial motion. The schema on the next page shows that, during flexion, the two components of this joint move in opposite directions like the teeth of two cogwheels:

- the basilar part of the occipital bone rises towards the vault with a very slight posterior displacement;
- while the basilar part of the sphenoid (the posterior part of the bone) also rises towards the vault, but with an anterior displacement.

During the normal movement of extension (the relaxation phase), these two components of the joint move passively in the inverse direction.

This displacement is responsible for pulling on the other bones during cranial motion, which is enhanced by the intrinsic plasticity of the bones.

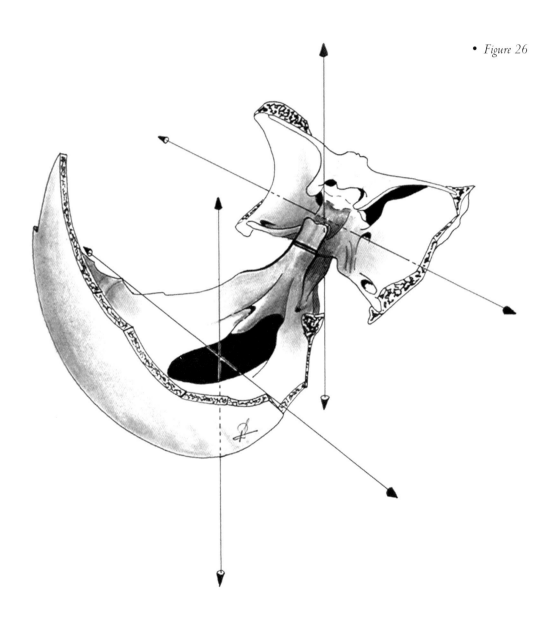

• *Figure 26*

Movement of the frontal bone

In cranial technique, the frontal bone is considered to consist of two parts because the metopic suture increases the plasticity of movement between the two bones that form its convex surface, and the bony lamellae, located between its three pillars (two lateral and one central), further enhance the plasticity of movement.

The main movement of the frontal bone occurs around a central axis and displaces its posterosuperior border both posteriorly and inferiorly, whereas the superciliary arches move anteriorly and superiorly.

At the same time, these structures also produce a slight depression of the metopic suture and an antero-lateral elevation of the two zygomatic processes.

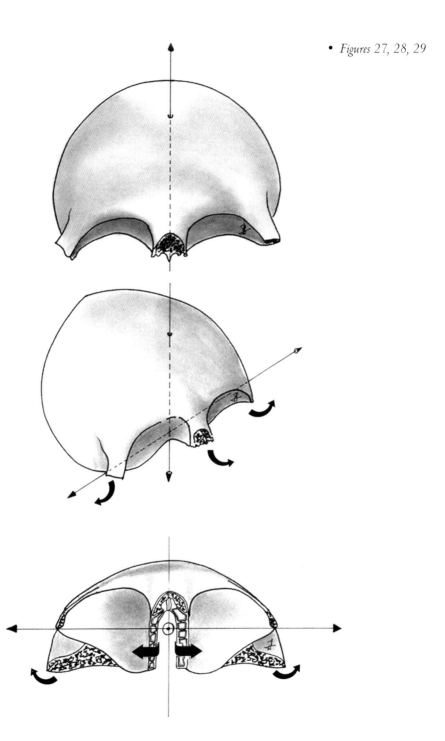

• *Figures 27, 28, 29*

Movement of the ethmoid

The ethmoid, which according to anatomists belongs either to the upper level of the cranium or to the face, contains lines of force that turn horizontal forces into vertical ones and vice versa. These movements are due to the stresses imposed on its central part; at the same time, its lateral parts contribute to the lateral expansion of the face as the maxillary bones rotate laterally.

Its transverse axis of rotation lies in the superior part of its perpendicular plate. Flexion about this axis is produced by the anterior part of the sphenoid, which pulls its posterior part inferiorly and laterally while its anterior part moves superiorly and posteriorly.

This movement corresponds exactly to that of the ethmoidal notch of the frontal bone, which contains the perpendicular plate of the ethmoid.

It is worth noting that both the plasticity of the bone and the fronto-ethmoidal suture allow small lateral movements as well as small adaptive and compensatory movements to occur.

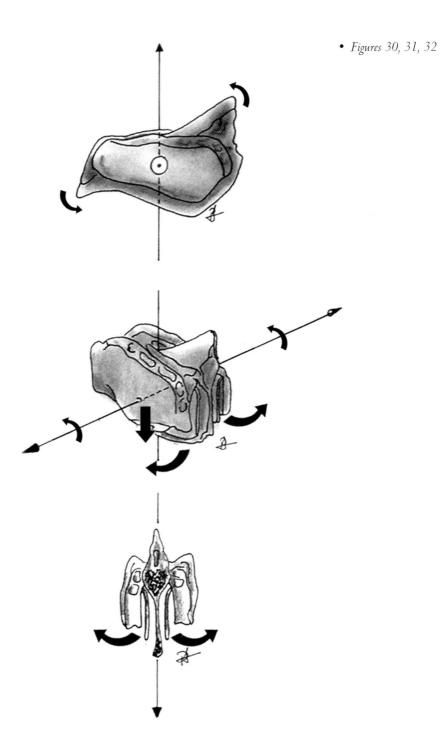

• *Figures 30, 31, 32*

Movement of the vomer

The vomer is a lamellar bone with oblique lines of force that run inferiorly and anteriorly; on the one hand, they balance vertical forces and, on the other, they stabilize the maxillary vault laterally.

This double role forces the bone to offset this double stress by undergoing torsion. The transverse axis of the vomer lies in its central part between the strongest lines of force.

The vomer is flexed by the action of the inferior part of the body of the sphenoid in such a way that its superior part moves inferiorly and anteriorly, while its inferior part moves inferiorly and posteriorly. These movements correspond exactly to the movements of the palatine processes of the maxillae and of the horizontal lamellae of the palatine bones.

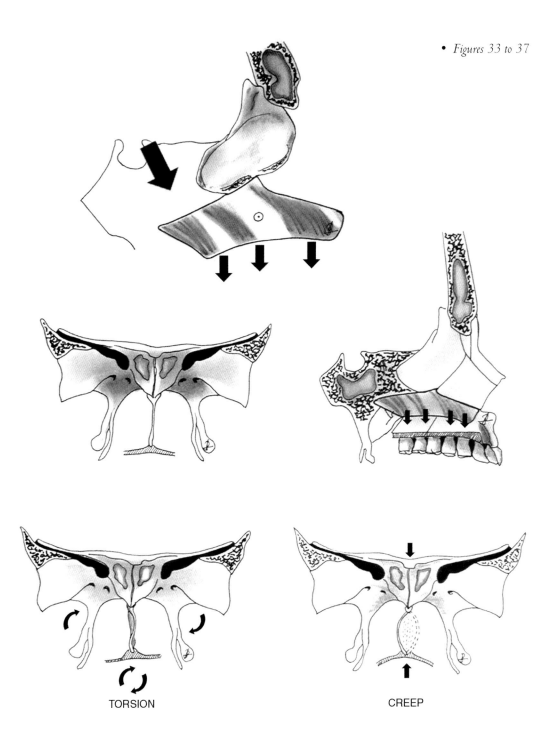

• *Figures 33 to 37*

TORSION

CREEP

Movements of the peripheral bones (the paired bones)

The cranial vault

The cranial vault combines:

- paired bones of membranous origin, such as the parietal bones;
- paired (temporal) and unpaired (occipital, frontal, and sphenoid) bones of mixed embryological origin:
  - membranous for the squamous components;
  - cartilaginous for the basilar components.

Its general structure, which is arched and plastic with well-developed lines of force, makes it supple and resistant.

Its accommodating dynamics are the result of its plasticity and of the significant movements that take place in the various types of sutures (denticulate, limbous, plane, etc.), which in turn allow small displacements to occur.

These bones lie at the edges of the cranial cavity, and all of them move about their axes with different degrees of obliquity.

Only one axis will be mentioned here for each movement described. This simple approach is for teaching purposes, and one must bear in mind that the axis of any movement changes direction as the movement proceeds and that these successive axes will describe a particular curve in space called the cardioid.

The coronal, lambdoid, and occipito-temporal sutures show a variable degree of beveling, which provides the pivots for the movements of each of the bones of the vault.

In fact, these pivots, gathered in a two-by-two arrangement, control the axes of movement of the parietal bones and of their articulations with the frontal bone and the occipital bone.

The movements of the paired peripheral bones, which take place about variable oblique axes, produce *external rotation* during their *phase of expansion* and *internal rotation* during the *relaxation phase*.

Let us look at the movements of these bones one by one.

Biomechanical features

The movements of the temporal bone are very complex and take place around three axes, which permit these movements to be spatially finely tuned.

In fact, the squamous and petrous parts of the temporal bone form two planes that intersect at about 90°. Each part has three pivots, around which each suture moves in a different way, allowing the bone to adopt an infinite number of orientations in space. The petrous part contains the three orthogonally arranged semicircular canals. The external auditory canal forms an angle of 10° with the occipital bone.

This resembles the mobility of the cervical column, the main goal of which is to ensure that vision is horizontal. The mobility of the temporal bone, which is as precise, would therefore allow this balancing system to be precisely spatially orientated so as to receive faithfully its afferent stimuli.

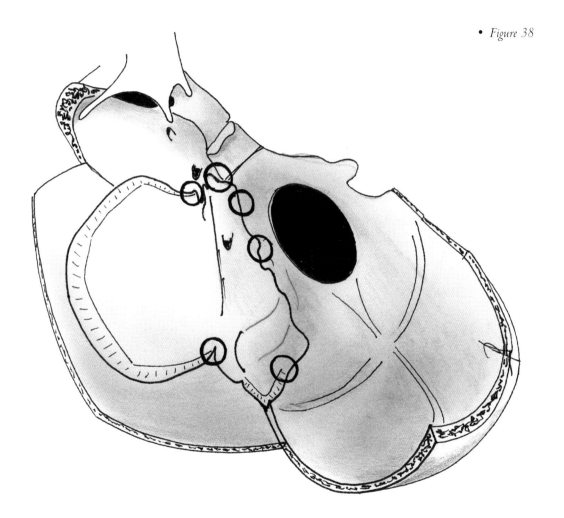

• Figure 38

Movement of the temporal bone

The axis of the temporal bone passes roughly through its pyramid-shaped petrous region and moves generally along a cardioid, just like the petrosal region itself.

This bone has six pivots gathered into two groups of three, which then form two nearly orthogonal intersecting planes. This arrangement allows the bone to move in a specific way at each of these pivots, depending on the specific structure of the different types of sutures involved. As a result, each of these pivots provides finer control of movement and offsets any small potential losses of mobility. The method of detection of these movements that we have developed will lead to the diagnosis and choice of specific techniques in order to restore the general motion of the temporal bone.

Let us first scrutinize the overall spectrum of movements of the temporal bone, which consists of four quite distinct sequences (see diagram on the next page) starting from its neutral position:

- external rotation;
- depression;
- extreme rotation;
- internal rotation.

• *Figures 39 to 42*

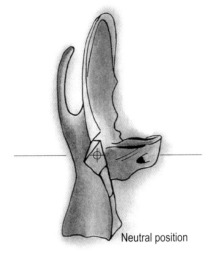

Neutral position

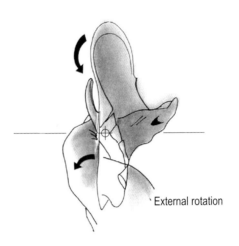

External rotation

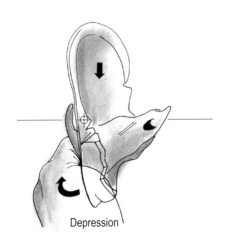

Depression

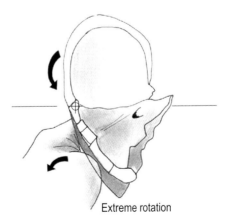

Extreme rotation

Movement of the pivots of the temporal bone

The three pivots of the cranial base

The petro-basilar pivot The articular surfaces involved include the seams located at the base of the occipital bone and the grooves lying in the temporal petrous, where it articulates with the occipital bone.

Its axis is transverse.

It undergoes a gliding movement that allows the cranium to expand.

The petro-jugular pivot The two articular surfaces make up the medial wall of the jugular foramen and, according to some anatomists, may contain a small meniscus.

Movement occurs about two axes: a transverse axis for external rotation and a vertical axis for clockwise rotation at the occipital level and anticlockwise rotation at the temporal level.

The spheno-petrous pivot Circumduction of the sphenoid takes place about the clinoid insertion of the *petro-sphenoid ligament (Grüber's ligament)*.

This movement stabilizes the structures forming the *cavernous sinus* and *the foramen lacerum*.

• *Figure 43*

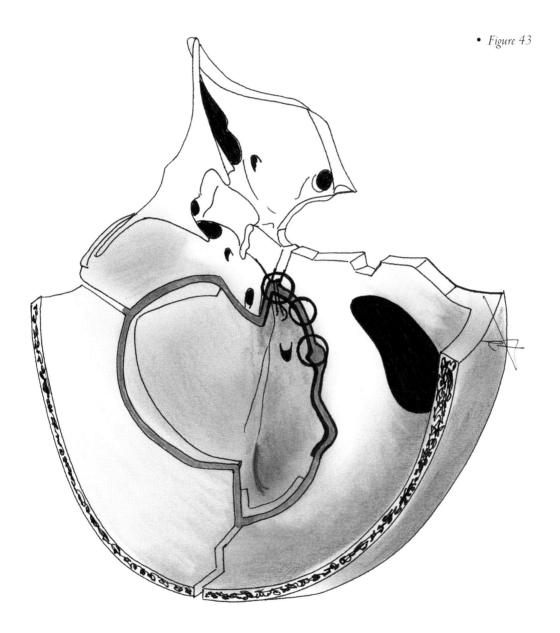

The three pivots of the vault

The condylo-squamo-mastoidal pivot This lies between the occipital and the posterior part of the mastoid at the point at which the beveling changes orientation from supero-medial to infero-lateral.

The temporal bone rotates externally on its transverse axis, while the pivot moves anteriorly about a vertical axis and away from the occipital bone.

The hinge–mastoid (HM) pivot This lies between the parietal and temporal bones at the point at which there is a slight change in orientation of the bevel of the temporal squama from lateral to medial (the *entomion*). This tiny change of beveling into a lateral orientation against a general background of medial orientation is responsible for a movement similar to that of a buckled wheel, such that the axis of the bone is lowered while increasing its *external rotation*.

This combination gives rise to the so-called *extreme rotation*.

The spheno-squamous pivot This lies between the posterior border of the greater wing of the sphenoid and the anterior border of the temporal squama, where the bevels of these two bones change in orientation with their inferior borders. The sphenoid moves around its three axes.

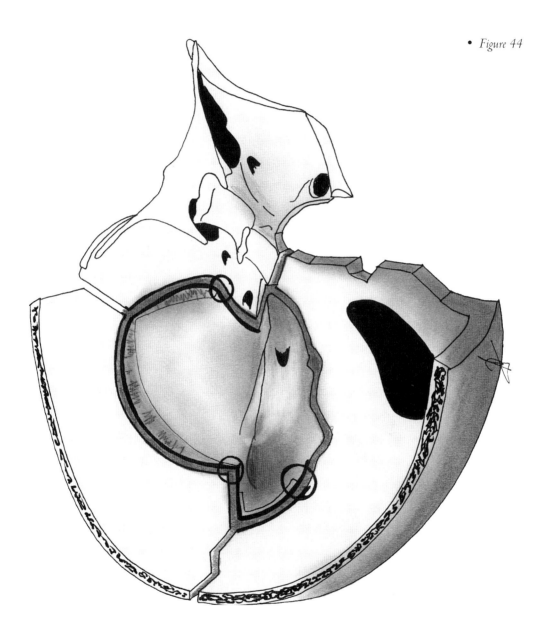

• *Figure 44*

Movement of the parietal bone

Its two sutures (i.e., the coronal and the lambdoid) contain two bevels, the lateral one being internal and the medial one external.

The pivot point lies where the bevels of these sutures change orientation. The two pivot points of the coronal and lambdoid sutures combine to form the axis of movement for each parietal bone.

At its squamous suture with the temporal squama, the parietal bone has an externally oriented bevel, except in the very tiny area of the HM pivot, where the orientation changes from external to internal.

The movements of the parietal bone can be summarized as follows.
During external rotation, which is synchronous with flexion of the unpaired bones:

- the antero-medial angle and the lateral part of the coronal suture move anteriorly and are everted;
- the medial part of the coronal suture sinks in and moves posteriorly, like the bregma;
- the sagittal suture sinks in and moves posteriorly while its two borders move apart, especially along its posterior part;
- the lambda sinks in and its two parietal borders move apart, while its occipital border moves posteriorly;
- the lambdoid suture sinks in and moves apart in its medial area, while its lateral area moves anteriorly and is everted;
- the temporal suture is everted and opened.

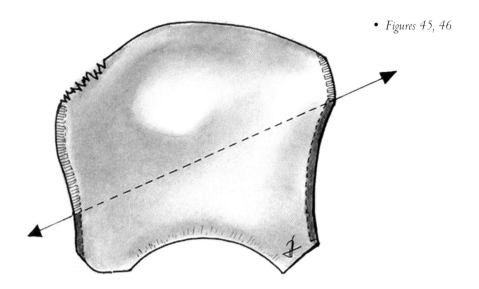

• *Figures 45, 46*

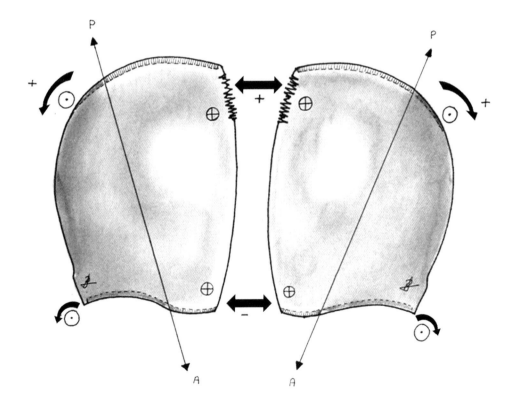

Movement of the facial bones

The sphenoid, temporal, and frontal bones transmit their movements to the maxilla, which interacts with them and transfers these movements to all of the bones that articulate with it (i.e., all the other bones of the face).

This is the moment of sutural opening.

While the slope of the forehead increases, the face widens as a whole and becomes more round. The eyes open. The mandible retreats and moves inferiorly.

The diagram on the opposite page illustrates the general movement of each facial bone. We shall now study the special features of each bone one by one.

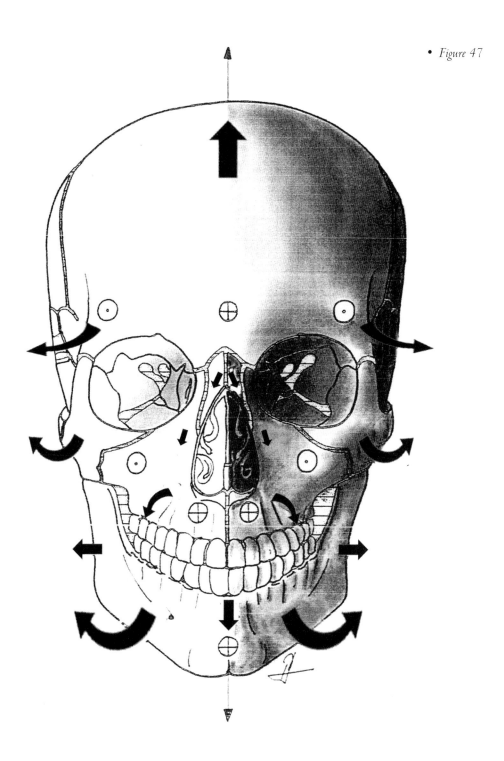

• *Figure 47*

Movement of the central maxillo-palatino-vomerian complex

This complex, as we have already noted, receives all of the radiating waves that result from direct shocks to the cranium. This is because it is the meeting point of the lines of force of the cranial architecture, i.e., its beams and pillars, which were identified long ago, notably by Felizet or Bennighoff, and also because it is continuous with the dura mater, which has been well described by Arbuckle.

We know that this complex must use its dynamic flexibility to respond to the intrinsic limitations of its bony environment, i.e., to the mechanical constraints imposed by the frontal and sphenoid bones.

It must therefore adapt its position to take into account the following small movements:

- spheno-maxillary torsion;
- shearing motion between the sphenoid and the maxilla;
- disengagement of the spheno-maxillary suture;
- lateral flexion of the fronto-maxillary suture;
- separation of the fronto-maxillary suture;
- antero-posterior shearing motion at the fronto-maxillary suture.

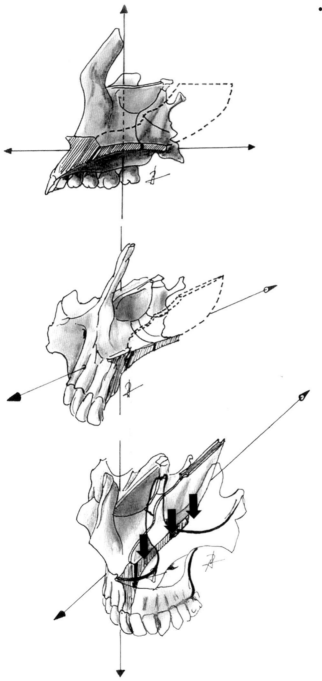

Movement of the maxilla

External–internal rotation of the maxilla takes place about an oblique axis that runs superiorly through its frontal process and inferiorly through its antero-lateral angle (i.e., the apex of its tuberosity).

Whereas the sphenoid flexes, each maxilla moves as if it were hanging from its frontal process and is displaced into a more coronal plane. The intermaxillary suture is lowered and moves posteriorly, and each maxilla appears to move away from the other posteriorly.

The posterior border of the frontal process rises and moves laterally so that it comes to lie in a more coronal plane, while its anterior aspect moves antero-laterally.

It is worth noting that the palatine process of each maxilla undergoes a movement parallel with and identical to that of the corresponding parietal bone.

As the two maxillary bones flex, the vault of the palate assumes a "romanesque" appearance, whereas, during extension, the vault is more like a Gothic arch.

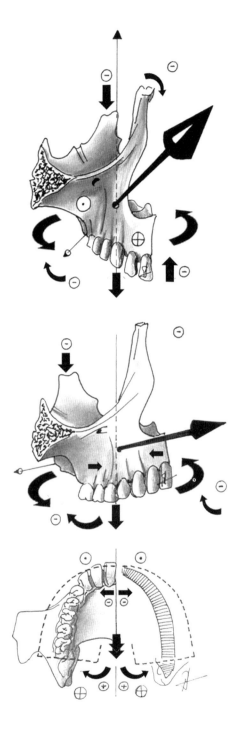

• *Figures 51, 52, 53*

Movement of the palatine bone

The structure of the palatine bone demonstrates its biomechanical role in cranial motion perfectly. It is formed by two flexible orthogonal planes, which meet to form a reinforced line of force running antero-posteriorly and which provide the requisite flexibility where the cranial system transforms horizontal forces into vertical forces and vice versa.

On one hand, its movement follows that of the pterygoid processes of the sphenoid, which support its sphenoidal process, and, on the other, it moves posteriorly following the movement of the maxillary palatine process, which supports its anterior border. Furthermore, its flexibility in the vertical plane allows it to offset the slightly oblique postero-lateral movement of the pterygoid processes.

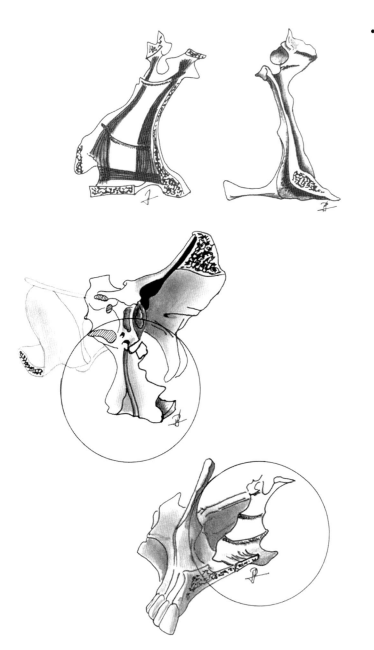

• *Figures 54 to 57*

Movement of the zygoma (the zygomatic process of the temporal bone)

The zygoma consists of dense and strong bone and articulates with the maxilla, frontal, and temporal bones.

Its oblique axis runs from a point located slightly below the glabella to the gonion. Hence, during flexion, the zygoma rotates antero-laterally, pulling its orbital border laterally and widening the orbit. Its frontal process follows the zygomatic process of the frontal bone and moves anteriorly and laterally, while its temporal process moves infero-laterally.

Movement of the nasal bone

The nasal bone articulates with the nasal spine of the frontal bone and follows its movements.

Its axis runs from its superior to its inferior border across its body in an oblique fashion inferiorly, anteriorly, and laterally.

During flexion, it rotates about this axis, while its central part is depressed and its peripheral part is elevated and everted.

Movement of the lacrimal bone

This lamellar bone, which is the size of a fingernail, moves slightly inferiorly, anteriorly, and laterally, thus deepening slightly the concavity of its internal surface.

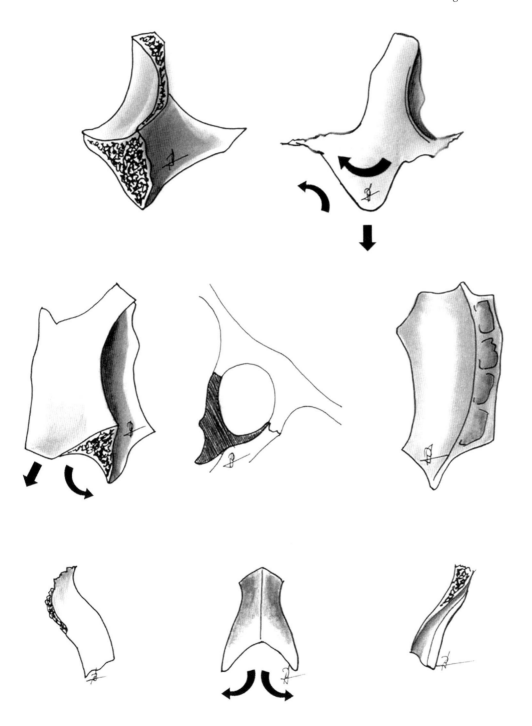

• *Figures 58 to 65*

Movement of the mandible

The mandible is the dependent part of the temporo-mandibular joint, and it is attached to the temporal bone by the collateral and stylo-mandibular ligaments and by its meniscus.

Therefore, its movement follows that of the portion of the temporal bone with which it is most closely associated (i.e., the mandibular fossa).

We know that, during external rotation, the part of the temporal bone that lies below its axis of rotation drops down, recedes, and moves slightly laterally. The mandible makes the same movement and also widens because of the structural capabilities of the symphysis menti.

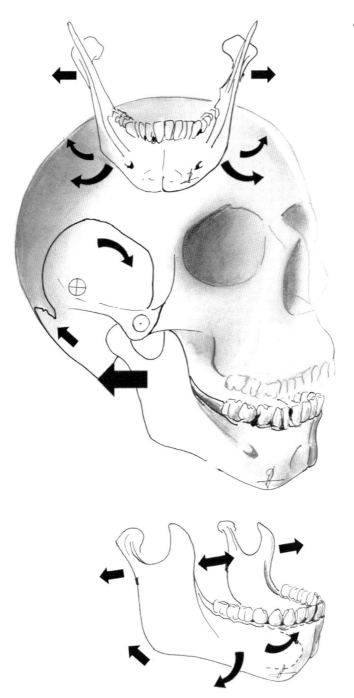

• *Figures 66, 67*

Movement of the reciprocal tension membranes

We shall concentrate on the purely biomechanical role of the *tentorium cerebelli*, which is a transverse partition dividing the cranial contents into two storeys, and of the *falx cerebri*, which is a mid-sagittal partition separating the two cerebral hemispheres.

Their superficial insertions consist of two layers, each attached either to the margin of a suture or to the border of a bony groove containing a venous sinus. Their deep insertions constitute a balance point (i.e., a flexible and variable fulcrum) at the level of the straight sinus. Thus, this membrane complex forms an internal balancing system for the cranium where the lines of force of the cranium and of the membranes become continuous and unite in order to distribute evenly the stresses imposed on the entire system.

The diagrams included on the following pages illustrate these lines of force, which can become lines of stress, as well as the movement of the tentorium cerebelli and of the falx cerebri during cranial flexion.

• *Figure 68*

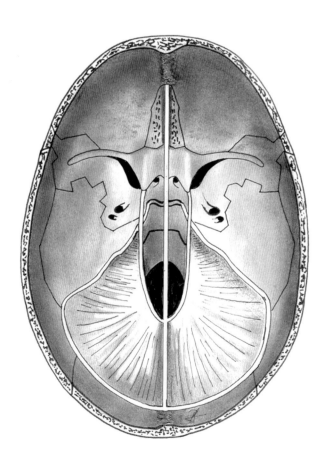

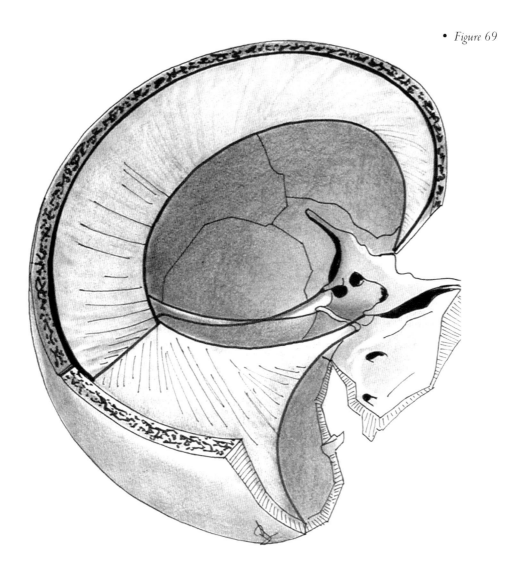

• *Figure 69*

• *Figure* 70

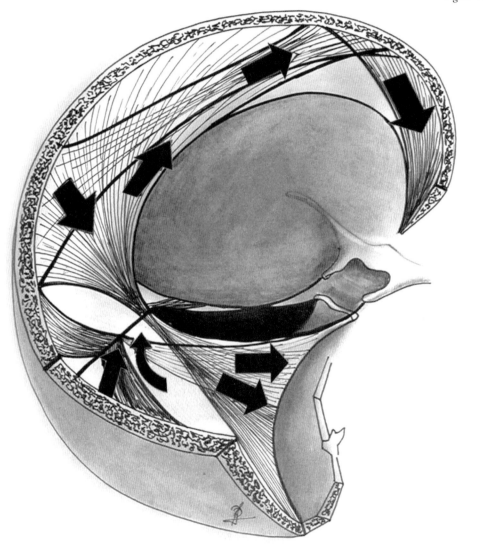

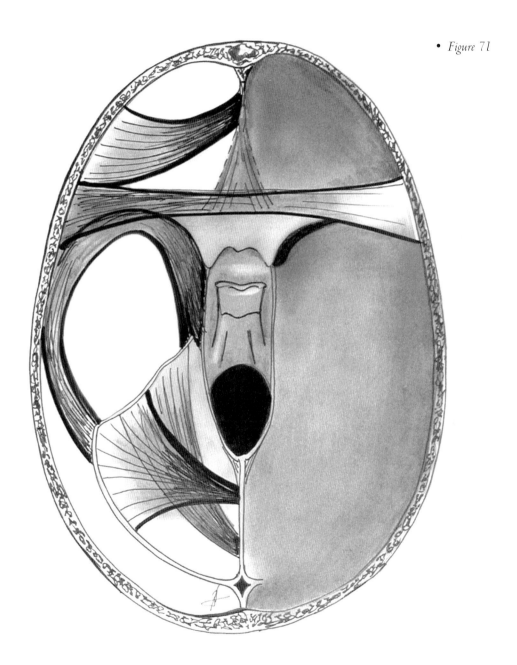

• *Figure 71*

Modes of cranial adaptation

The development of cranial adaptation

Humans fail to maintain their potential for functional freedom throughout life because age progressively alters its structural basis. Points of reduced or null mobility develop here and there as a result of certain postures, dysfunctions, traumas, gestures imperfectly performed, and of muscular or fascial tensions (or both) created by an individual's emotional reactions to life experiences.

This partial loss of freedom will sporadically restrict functional activity and will lead to more or less permanent muscular or fascial tensions, or both, that will influence the subject's general performance and, at the same time, impart certain characteristics to his or her body language. It is a biological law that humans, regardless of acquired restraints, seek to live their lives as fully as possible by using typical modes of adaptation that allow them to function to the maximum of their residual capabilities.

Torsion is the first stage of our adaptation

As we have shown elsewhere, the first stage of this adaptation uses torsion, as this position allows the body to maintain its full functional potential, and even to enhance it, for two reasons. First, the continuous fascial system that spans our entire body allows us to become taller by unwinding from a fixed point (i.e., the ground) while keeping our balance. (This is demonstrated very well by the person who twists as he stretches to unscrew a light bulb that he could not have touched before.)

Second, this position allows us to store the *potential energy* gained during the movement of extension, which the body will then pay back as *kinetic energy* on leaving this position. Such examples abound in sports: for example, the preliminary torsion needed for a backhand in tennis and for a return kick in football. The body has grasped the problem well. It tries to prevent a fall and will attempt to control it by acquiring additional kinetic energy as a result of torsion.

Rotation/lateral flexion is generally an extension of torsion

If torsion turns out to be inadequate, the body increases its internal stress by creating a fixed point from which a new balance will develop that will enable it to function. Unfortunately, this strategy is associated with the most severe functional restriction, again in accordance with the same biological law of functional survival.

Like every other subsystem of the human body, the cranium is subject to these laws. Thus, it begins by adopting the position of torsion in order to go on functioning almost normally. Then, if this fails, it develops a less mobile zone of adaptation, which can follow a trauma whose wave of dispersion has overloaded the cranial system. Adaptation then occurs via rotation/lateral flexion.

This zone of cranial adaptation leads to the loss of some biomechanical capabilities and to a concurrent drop in intracranial blood flow, which results in a decrease in the much needed oxygen and glucose supply to the brain. Still in accordance with the same biological law, the body adopts the best solution to ensure its normal function in terms of continuity of life and survival.

Other forms of adaptation can occur, but they are secondary to stresses that occur very early in life – shortly after birth – and do not form part of the mechanism of general adaptation.

These are found in some small children, adolescents, or adults, and we shall outline the modes of adaptation most frequently encountered. They take place at the spheno-basilar synchondrosis. The main ones are:

- horizontal displacements;
- vertical displacements;
- compressive stresses.

The different modes of adaptation

Torsion

During flexion, each of the midline bones rotates around its transverse axis, while the peripheral bones rotate externally around their individual oblique axes.

Because of its central position, the spheno-basilar synchondrosis is the point of convergence of all the sutures of the cranial base, which mimic converging rays. It is very easy to understand that any restriction at one or more of these sutures will alter the movement of flexion/external rotation around the new fixed point. A hinge is formed, forcing the cranial system to use another axis to complete the movement.

This new antero-posterior axis entails an additional movement of torsion with the anterior and posterior parts of the cranium moving in opposite directions. In addition, the plastic deformation of the cranium leads to a very small additional passive movement, which takes place around vertical axes and in the opposite direction.

This torsion is labeled "*right-sided*" or "*left-sided*" depending on the side where the greater wing of the sphenoid reaches a higher position vertically while it turns slightly towards the opposite side.

Likewise, a vault suture that has exceeded its biomechanical capabilities of adaptation will create a fixed point of restriction at the cranial base, forcing the cranial system to undergo torsion in order to allow it to open up and expand rhythmically. Because of its basic plasticity, on the one hand, and the slight play occurring at the sutures, on the other, the cranial complex can normally adapt in torsion depending on the mechanical constraints that are placed upon it during daily activities.

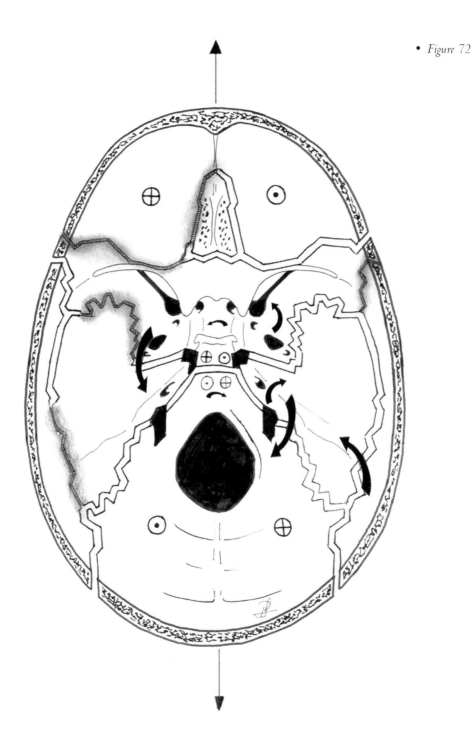

• *Figure 72*

• *Figure 73*

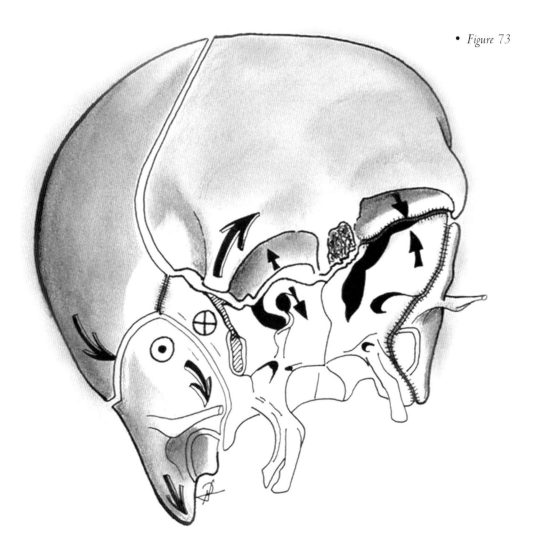

For this reason, detection of this capability provides a precise test for the adaptability of the cranial system, especially as any type of interference with its motion reveals the state of its connective tissues.

The different modes of torsion illustrated here stress the anatomical locations that are particularly restricted during torsion.

When one of these sites of restricted movement becomes abnormally permanent, the cranium expands by undergoing torsion, as we have just seen, in order to complete its movement of flexion/expansion, which is its *raison d'être*.

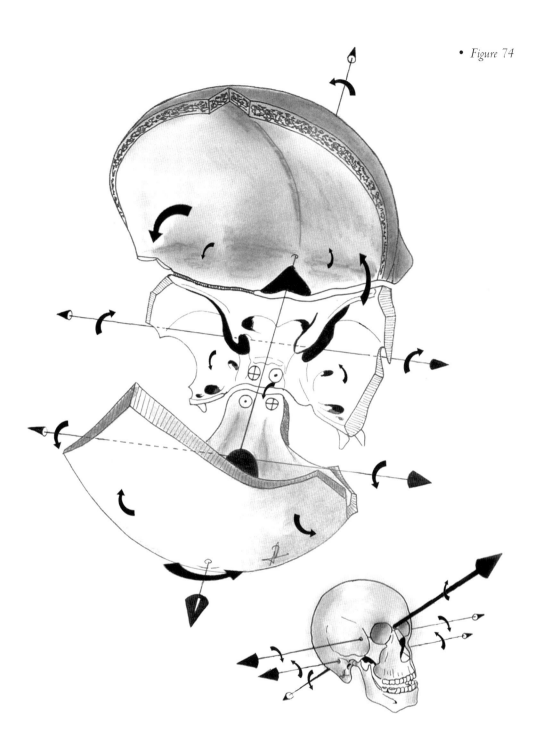

• *Figure 74*

It is the role of the therapist to perform manual tests in order to determine precisely any loss or alteration of function (*dysfunction*) and thus to establish the nature of the restriction. Thus, the therapist can choose the most suitable treatment modalities and offer treatment appropriate to the findings. The quality of the final phase of the movement (*end feel of motion* for American authors, i.e., elasticity, resilience, etc.) will indicate whether or not it is normal. If it is not normal, it is advisable to take account of this restriction when the movement is induced or even slightly amplified by the therapist. The achievement of this movement is a diagnostic test.

• *Figure 75*

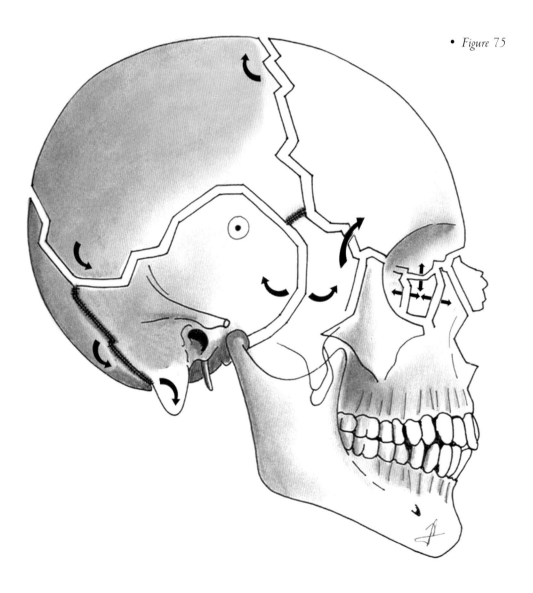

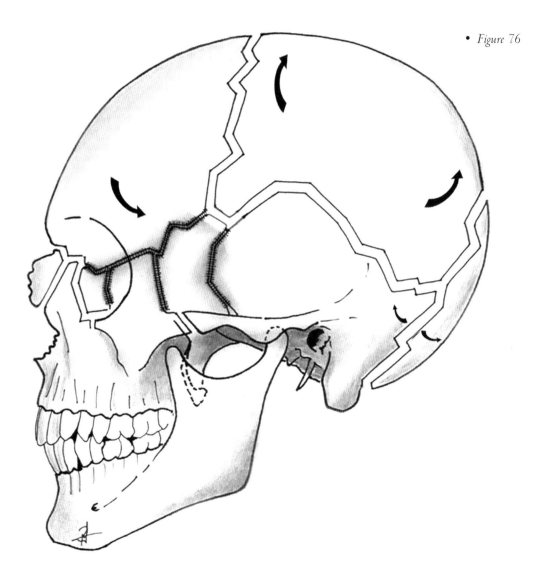

• *Figure 76*

Rotation/lateral flexion

When a stress exceeds the cranial system's ability to undergo torsion, a different mode of adaptation comes into play that allows the forces to be dispersed in a new way by providing an additional compensatory pathway in the third spatial dimension. But in so doing, it creates a new zone of functional restriction.

This is *rotation/lateral flexion* associated with the following:

- flexion around the transverse axes;
- lateral inclination of the entire cranium about an antero-posterior axis;
- rotation in the opposite direction of the anterior and posterior halves of the cranium around two vertical axes that run through the body of the sphenoid and occipital bones.

This is labeled according to the side on which the spheno-basilar synchondrosis opens up.

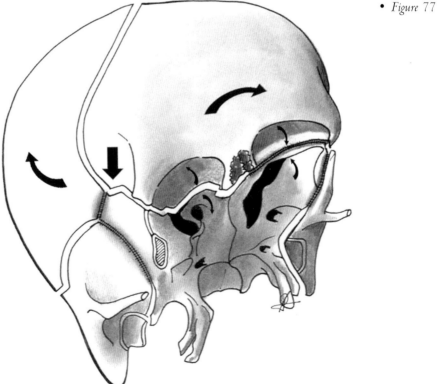

• *Figure 77*

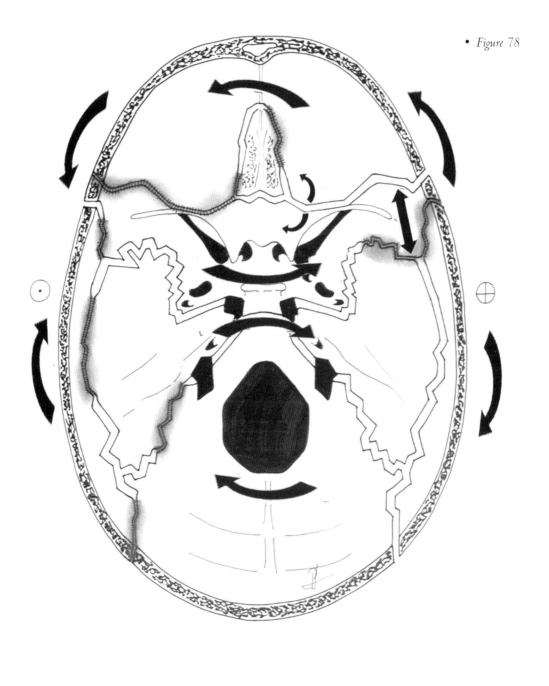

• *Figure 78*

We have seen that, as a result of its basic plasticity and the small degree of play at its sutural articulations, the cranial complex can normally adapt to any stress imposed during rotation/lateral flexion. Hence, during diagnostic tests, the therapist takes the cranial complex through this pathway of adaptation in order to verify freedom of movement at the sutures as well as to check the condition of the connective tissues.

The quality of the final phase of the movement (i.e., its elasticity and its resilience) will identify structural normality or a *cranial osteopathic lesion* in one of the restriction points caused by the stress, illustrated by the diagrams on the opposite page as well as on the two previous pages.

We have seen that, when the human body falls and is unable to right itself, it automatically tries to increase its coefficient of dispersion of stresses in anticipation of the forthcoming shock by enhancing the pliability of the part of the body that will bear the brunt of the shock and absorb it. It does this by making use appropriately and naturally of its *tensegrity*, which we have already shown elsewhere, as follows:

- by increasing the elasticity of the side exposed to the shock wave (the contact side);
- by reinforcing the rigid components of the opposite side.

Thus, the stress imposed on the whole body is absorbed in the best way.
In the cranial system, every stress that exceeds its absorption capabilities through torsion will bring about a rotation/lateral flexion accompanied by compensatory functional losses on the opposite side, as shown previously.

The diagrams on the opposite page and on the next two pages illustrate the locations of the structural restrictions that are associated with this mode of adaptation.

• *Figure 79*

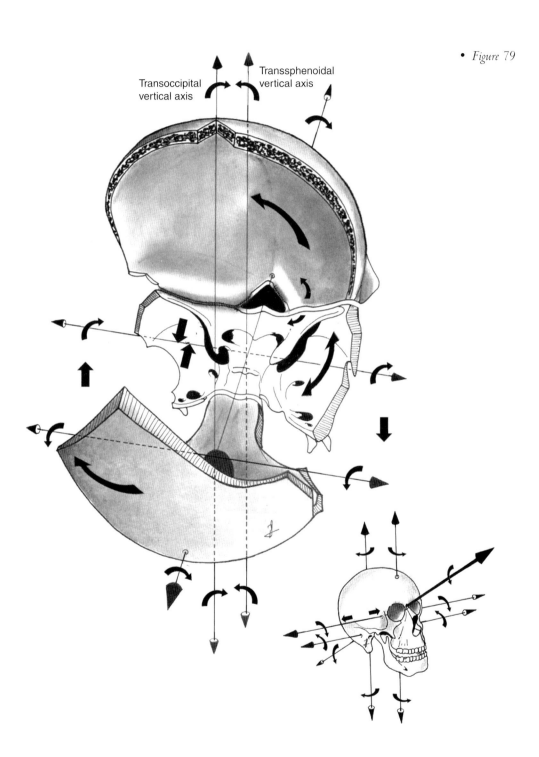

Transoccipital
vertical axis

Transsphenoidal
vertical axis

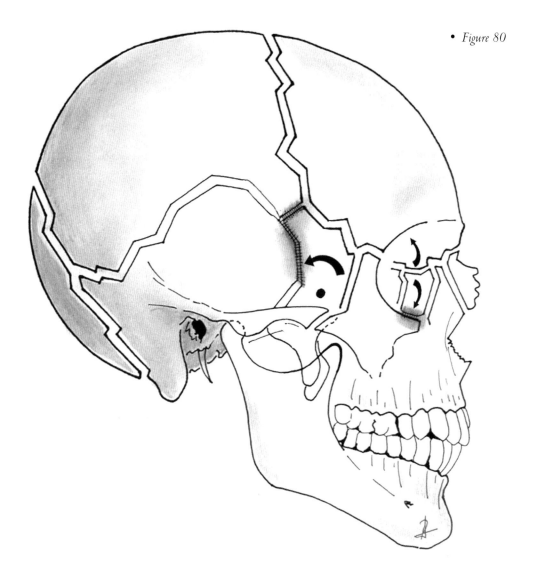

• *Figure 80*

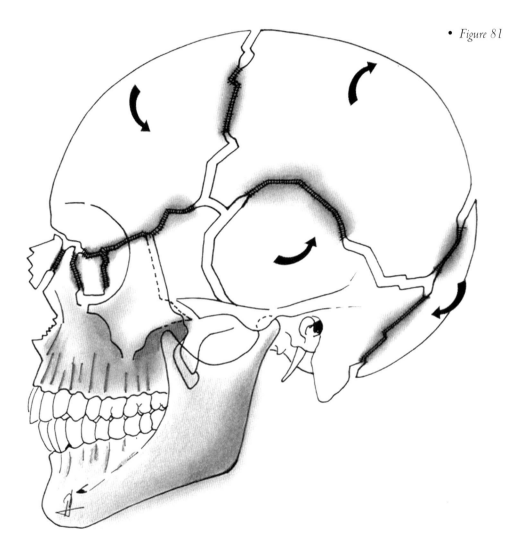

• *Figure 81*

Vertical upward displacement

This mode of adaptation is generally established very early on in cranial development when the sutures are not yet dovetailed but are still made up of two distinct bones side by side, and when the spheno-basilar synchondrosis still consists of two distinct bones. The equilibrium of the cranial system depends on its membranes and also on its own structural mass.

This displacement is the result of a stress that exceeds the adaptive capabilities of the cranial system as defined by its flexibility and its plasticity.
Its anterior and posterior parts are rotated around their respective transverse axes in opposite directions.

During vertical upward displacements, the midline bones of the cranial base move as follows:

• the sphenoid bone, and the other bones functionally under its control, move into flexion;

• the occipital bone and its satellites move into extension synchronously.

The sutural consequences are shown in the adjoining diagram and in the one on the next page.

• *Figure 82*

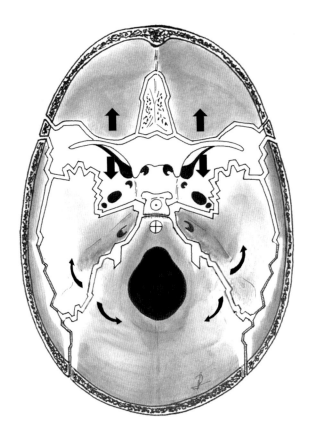

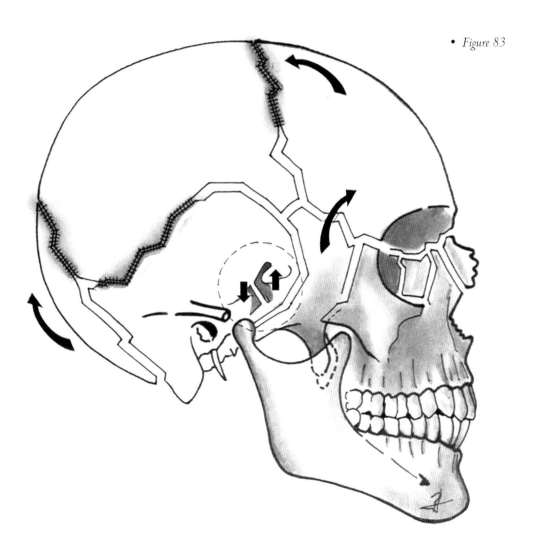

• *Figure 83*

We have seen that the cranial system with its structural plasticity and the slight degree of play at the sutures can normally adapt to all stresses developed during *vertical upward displacements*.

For this reason, in the course of diagnostic tests, the therapist takes the cranial system along this mode of adaptation in order to verify freedom of movement at the sutures as well as the condition of the connective tissues.

The quality of the final phase of the movement (i.e., its elasticity and resilience) will identify structural normality or a *cranial osteopathic lesion* at one of the points of restriction caused by that stress, as illustrated by the diagrams on the opposite page and on the two previous pages.

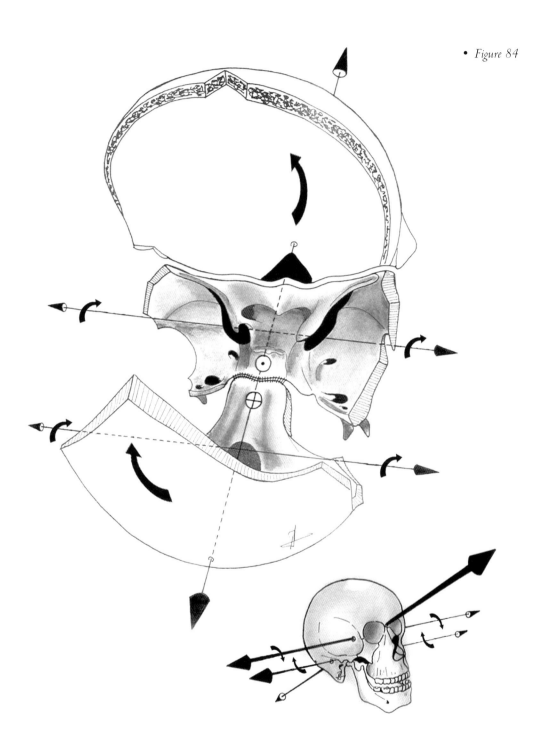

• *Figure 84*

Vertical downward displacement

This is the exact opposite of the previous displacement. Thus, the following movements take place about the same respective transverse axes in the midline bones of the cranial base:

- the sphenoid bone, and its functionally dependent bones, move into extension;
- the occipital bone and its satellites move into flexion.

It is obvious that all the peripheral bones of the cranium and the facial bones will adapt, as illustrated by the diagrams below and on the opposite page. Also shown are the various effects of these stresses on each suture.

• *Figure 85*

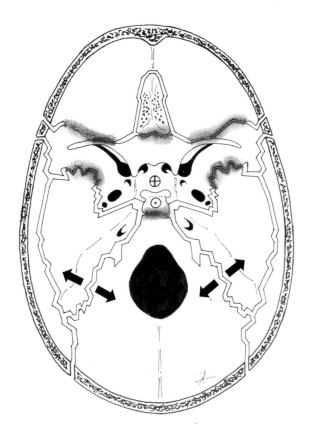

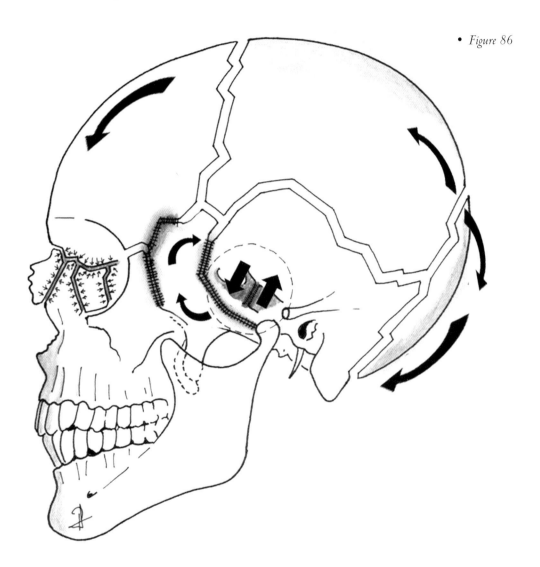

• *Figure 86*

We have seen that the entire cranial system, with its structural plasticity and a slight degree of play at the sutures, can also normally adapt to all stresses generated during a *vertical downward displacement*.

For this reason, in the course of diagnostic tests, the therapist should take the cranial system along that mode of adaptation in order to verify freedom of movement at the sutures as well as the condition of their connective tissues.

The quality of the final phase of the movement (i.e., its elasticity and resilience) will identify structural normality or a *cranial osteopathic lesion* at one of the points of restriction caused by that stress, as illustrated in the diagram on the opposite page and in those on the two preceding pages.

• *Figure* 87

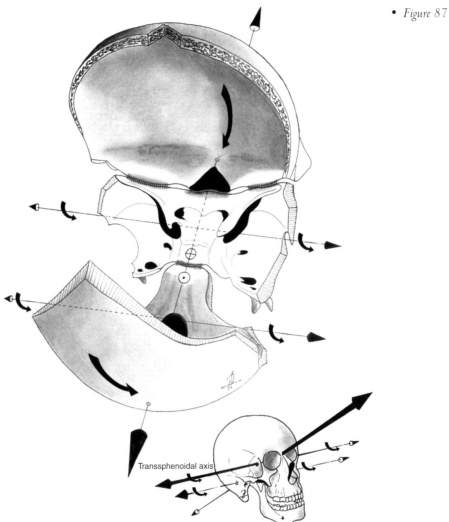

Transsphenoidal axis

Lateral displacement

Just like the modes of adaptation mentioned above, that involving *lateral displacement* takes place very early on in cranial development. Lateral displacement is the result of a stress that exceeds the adaptive capabilities of the cranium (i.e., its pliability and plasticity) and is applied from the side in this case.

The anterior and posterior parts of the cranium at the level of the midline bones of the cranial base are displaced in the same direction during the expansion phase, as follows:

• the sphenoid bone, and the bones that are moved by it, rotate about a vertical axis running through the body of the sphenoid;

• the occipital bone and its satellites are displaced in the same direction about an axis passing through its body.

These movements appear to open the spheno-basilar synchondrosis on the side opposite the direction of torsion, and the displacement is labeled according to the side involved.

As described previously, during evaluation the cranial mechanism must be able, if it is free, to adapt to the movement initiated by the practitioner's fingers. Inability to induce this movement indicates sutural restrictions, the anatomical locations of which are indicated in the diagrams on the following pages.

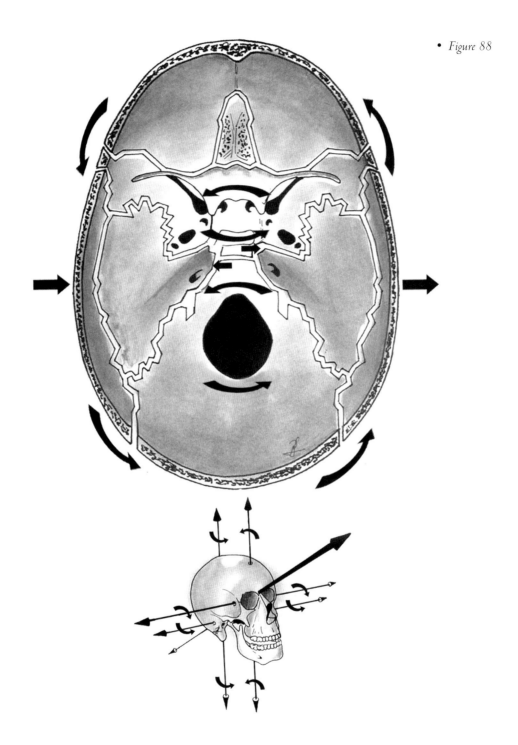

• *Figure 88*

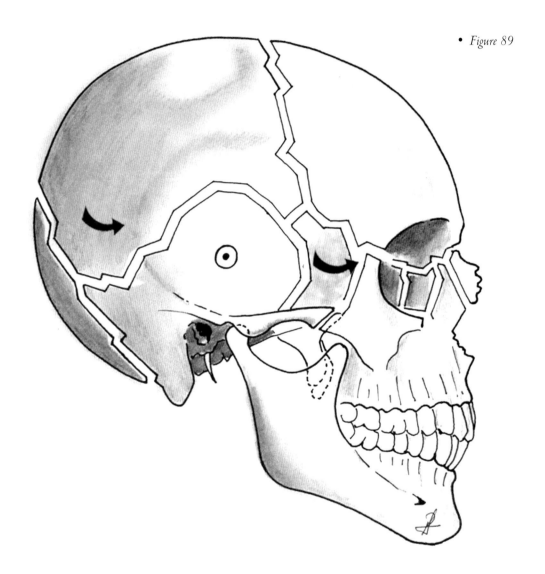

• *Figure 89*

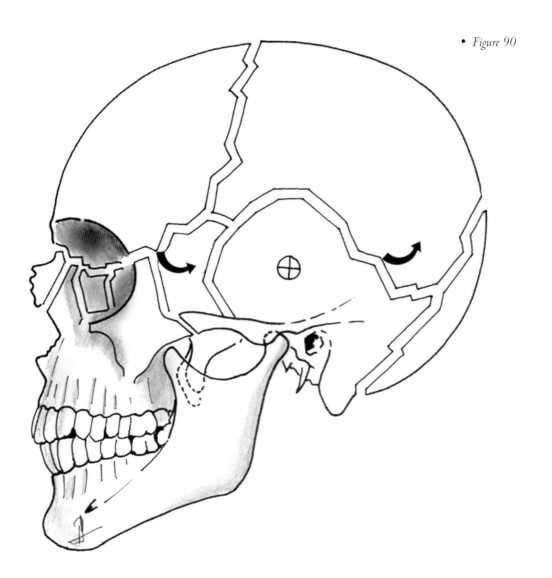

• *Figure 90*

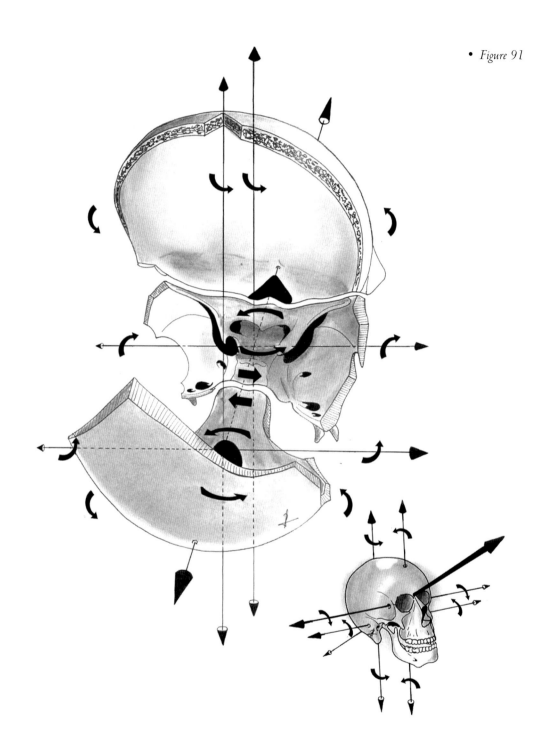

• *Figure 91*

PART TWO

Pathomechanics

The cranial osteopathic lesion

Tissue changes are caused by biomechanical disturbances that result from uncompensated changes in the blood supply, in the levels of blood-borne hormones, and/or in neural control. They equate to a loss of water content that results in changes in the plasticity and elasticity of normal tissues and that produces *a fixed point* within these tissues.

This new fixed point is the osteopathic lesion.

We insist that "fixed point" does not mean "immobile point," but that it signifies a fixed point with respect to the intrinsic dynamic properties of the tissue under consideration (i.e., a point of reduced mobility in terms of its normal movement potential).

Physical features of the osteopathic lesion

- Change in tissue characteristics:
  - reduced plasticity;
  - reduced elasticity.
- Reduced mobility.
- Loss of end-of-movement elasticity with a clear-cut cessation of movement (abrupt and without any smoothness).
- The joint is unable to store the terminal component of the kinetic energy of movement, which is released when the joint returns to the neutral position and is a usual characteristic of joint flexibility.
- Pain reflecting tissue damage.

- As each bone is related to at least two joints, any change will be transmitted to at least those two joints, with the result that the second joint will undergo a similar movement to the first (i.e., *synkinesis*). In other words, movement at the proximal joint is altered by the movement taking place at the abnormal joint.

We can see right away that these changes demonstrate an osteopathic lesion that we can feel with our fingers as:

- changes in the nature of the tissues;
- reduced mobility with an abrupt cessation at the end of a normal movement;
- pain to the touch;
- synkinesis.

These signs will establish the clinical picture and permit the diagnosis of the osteopathic lesion.

Osteopathic diagnosis

- Testing the degree of tissue resistance to evaluate the tissue changes.
- Dynamic testing to measure the flexibility at the end of a movement.
- Palpation of the abnormal tissues to assess the damage.
- Testing the proximal joints to measure the degree of functional impairment.

It is clear that the cranial osteopathic approach will have to follow the same process, i.e., the same diagnostic approach, the same search for objective physical signs revealing the lesion, and, finally, the same rational approach to the choice of therapeutic modalities.

Synopsis of osteopathic practice

Pathogenesis

Biomechanical pathogenetic factors include:

- local factors;
- disturbances in control mechanisms;
- abnormalities in functional links.

Vasculo-humoral pathogenetic factors include:

- local factors;
- disturbances in control mechanisms;
- remote abnormalities.

Neurological pathogenetic factors include:

- local factors;
- disturbances in control mechanisms;
- remote abnormalities.

These signs, which reveal the lesion, will allow the osteopathic diagnosis to be made and will lead the practitioner to formulate the proper therapeutic conclusions.

Therapeutic conclusions

- Establishing a therapeutic protocol based on the most appropriate diagnostic procedures.
- Defining the modalities for each technique:
  - contact point;
  - direction of movement during manipulation;
  - modalities of manipulation, such as speed, strength, etc.

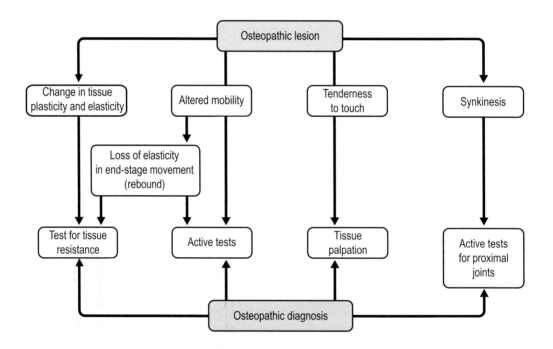

Reduction of the lesion

Once the restriction barrier is identified, we can evaluate its features, and this also allows us to choose the appropriate mode of treatment.

There are three possibilities:

The inductive technique

The therapist positions himself or herself against the site of the barrier, presses against it without increasing the pressure, and waits for the spontaneous release of the barrier.

Progressive reduction

The therapist's manipulation progressively permeates the lesion, an action that we represent in the form of a triangle of functional impairment in the range of movements at the joint. As the manipulation is repeated, the size of this triangle of weakness is partly reduced, signifying a progressive improvement in the barrier.

Thrust

The barrier is taken by surprise by the increasing pressure applied by the therapist, and it breaks down of its own accord.

Certainly, in this case, the type of manipulation chosen should vary in strength and speed in order to match perfectly the type and state of the tissue.

The choice of manipulation must also take into account another criterion, that of the neural background of the lesion. In our view, this gives rise to one of the main differences between a structural and a functional lesion.

Relevance to cranial lesions

Cranial articulation, as we have defined it (see p. 28), and its biomechanics (see p. 39) provide us with proof that the cranial system and every other joint in the body are functionally identical. It is therefore easy to grasp why the cranial system falls within the framework of osteopathy and why its lesions are similar to those of other joints.

The approach of the osteopathic practitioner will therefore be the same. Diagnosis consists of identifying the systems involved along with their lesions and noting the physical signs, which the practitioner will classify and organize rationally. The practitioner will then be able to choose the most appropriate therapy and the techniques to apply in accordance with the nature of the barrier and of the tissues involved.

In this context, a thorough knowledge of anatomy will be one of the essential pillars of the diagnostic procedure. It takes into account the patient's complaints and the functional and structural changes present, it links the physical signs to the underlying system involved, and it incorporates remote regulatory subsystems.

Of course, biomechanics is the second indispensable theoretical underpinning of the diagnostic procedure. It explains and gives meaning to whatever our hands feel. It also allows us to initiate a test to evaluate dysfunction and to perform a manipulation that determines the type of restriction and its attendant functional impairment.

The lesions of the cranial system have the same features as those of any other articulation:

- tissue changes with loss of plasticity, indicated by the loss of rebound at the end of a movement and the presence of elasticity only in the neutral phase of a movement during return to the neutral point;
- reduced mobility;
- occasional pain in the tissue;
- articular synkinesis, which can alter the normal relationship between bones.

Diagnosis is achieved by the usual method:

- palpation of the tissues of the suture;
- testing for tissue resistance, which allows a qualitative and quantitative assessment of the barrier (the rebound at the end of the movement);
- dynamic tests of function;
- tests using the movements of cranial adaptation to emphasize sutural restrictions.

PART THREE:

The Therapeutic Tools

The therapist's posture in cranial osteopathic technique

While touching the patient's head, the practitioner's hands must have no fixed point. This is to prevent any change to or limitation of the patient's cranial motion resulting from the contact.

Total freedom of cranial motion in the practitioner's hands eliminates the far too common interface between patient and practitioner and enables the latter to enjoy a range of perception extending at least to his or her abdomen.

To be as one with their patients, and to feel all their movements, therapists will eliminate any interface between themselves and their patients, thus creating a new kind of active interface that is remote from the physical setting. (The therapist sits on a chair with feet on the floor and the back of his or her hand resting on the table.)

The concept of the interface

The wind hits the sail and allows the boat to move. The sail is the point of energy transfer. Every interface needs an absolute intimacy of contact and interpenetration to transfer energy faithfully into a perfectly graded action.

Energy is like a wave that simultaneously transmits its force and its motion.

During therapy, the practitioner's hand blends intimately with the part of the body it is activating, and transmits to it the energy generated by its movement. To avoid breaking this union between hand and cranium, an interface is created between the back of the practitioner's hand and the treatment table (i.e., between the hand and the supporting surface on which it is moving).

It would be a mistake to create this interface between the palm of the hand and the cranium it is activating, as the energy would be partly dissipated.

To prevent this from happening, the practitioner very slightly increases the contact between hand and table, and thus indirectly enhances the harmony between hand and cranium.

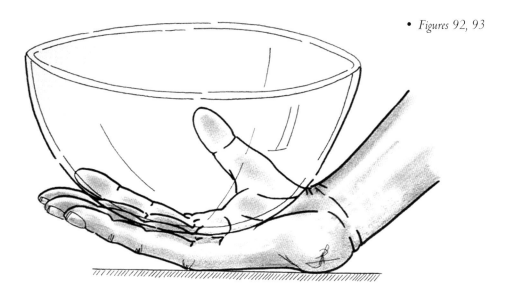

• *Figures 92, 93*

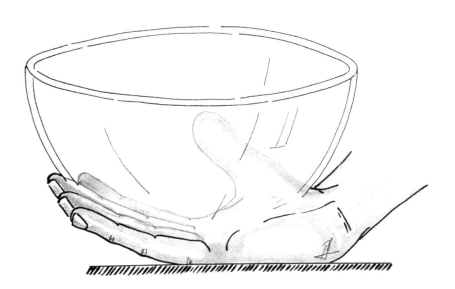

The concept of the fulcrum

Our concept is in keeping with the wider meaning given in the Heritage Dictionary: *a balance point, a position, element or action through, around and by means of which vital forces are exercised*. Our therapeutic action effectively combines all these aspects.

Therapists will create a new point of support exactly at the interface between the energy they are providing and the structure they wish to activate. Thus, they can focus their action precisely where necessary in order to feel the presence or absence of functional freedom of movement and to help them later to restore that freedom.

To act specifically on the tissue concerned, they will position their contact point at a suitable depth by using the density and presence of their hand and by relying on their own perception until the appropriate level is reached.

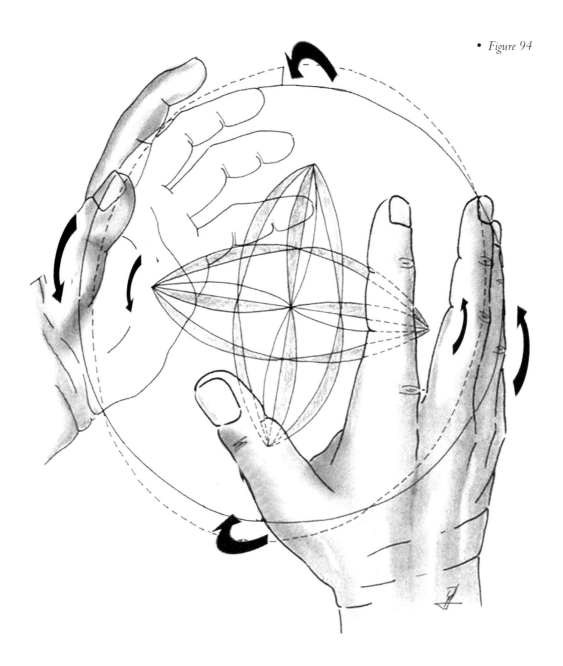

• *Figure 94*

Therapeutic palpation

Different forms of palpation are used in therapy, each of which has its own characteristics. These allow the therapist to establish a suitable relationship with the patient, to modulate a sensation, or to carry out a specific action. Therapists can therefore do the following:

- Make contact with the patient while maintaining a distinct boundary between themselves and the patient.

- Establish the same contact that is adopted in more intimate relationships, which removes any boundary between two people. (This is contact by "fusion." Let us remember the physical pain we feel when we are separated from a loved one.)

- Choose the "transference" mode, which is similar to the contact achieved in hand-shaking.

The last two forms of palpation do not involve a distinct boundary between the two people. In cranial therapy, we adopt a sociable form of palpation as follows:

- The pressure exerted is equal to the resistance of the tissue touched, thus eliminating the interface between practitioner and patient. (This is easily achieved, as we have seen, by transferring the interface to a point between the back of the therapist's hand, which is not in contact with the patient, and the surface of the treatment table.)

- The practitioner projects his or her perception on to this same level.

A perfect relationship is then created between these two people: every movement coming from the patient operates specifically at this same level.

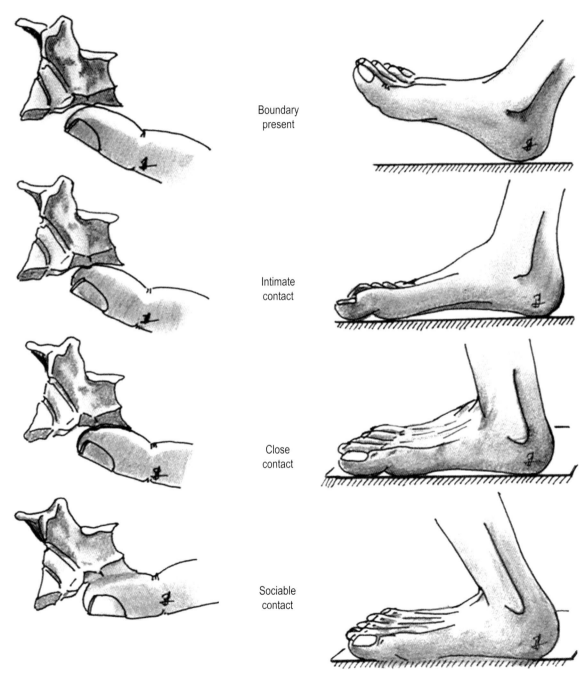

• *Figure 95*

Boundary present

Intimate contact

Close contact

Sociable contact

Symbiosis between patient and therapist: "the art of uniting and separating"

To illustrate the relationship between patient and therapist, one could picture two donkeys walking together along the crest of a narrow ridge. As the path is narrow, they lean against each other, which instinctively reassures them. When the terrain is less safe, the donkey on the outside leans more strongly on the other, which naturally reacts to this pressure. But if, depending on the hazards of the road, the donkey on the outside loses its footing, it will lean even further on its neighbor, which is walking on stable ground.

These donkeys are in a state of reciprocity and cooperation, which allows them to form a "tensegrity" unit. There is no interface between them, but they keep establishing a dynamic interface as they go along.

The same applies to the symbiosis between patient and therapist when the practitioner's hand eliminates the interface between his or her palm and the patient in order to create it elsewhere, and when it follows perfectly the reactions of the patient's cranium to the tests and treatments that are being applied.

• *Figure 96*

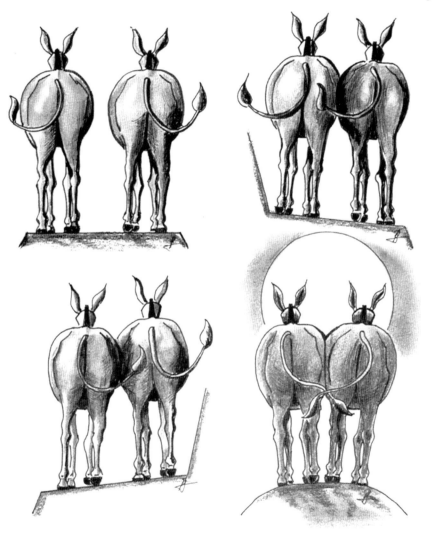

PART FOUR

Manual Diagnosis

Whichever technique is chosen, the approach to manual diagnosis in cranial therapy requires that the patient lie down comfortably on the treatment table in the supine position. The practitioner stands at the level of the patient's head. The general principles shared by various approaches are as follows:

- To establish contact, the practitioner uses the cooperative or reciprocal mode of palpation, which occurs naturally or is achieved by creating a very thin interface between the back of his or her hand and the surface of the treatment table.

- The practitioner then initiates each test by small movements of the body and evaluates the final rebound of each movement as well as the capacity of the cranial mechanism to adapt to its compensatory movements (torsion, rotation/lateral flexion, etc.).

- When in doubt, the practitioner can then add a final impulse at the end of the movement, which will allow him or her to feel the end-of-movement passive elasticity that every healthy articulation retains.

Manual approaches

The vault approach

This classic approach is the one chosen most often by practitioners because it allows them to feel the general motion of the cranial bones and the motion of a particular bone within the cranial system, and also to feel the freedom of movement at the spheno-basilar synchondrosis.

The fingers of both hands are spread out without any tension and form a cup designed to receive the very irregular convexity of the lateral, posterior, and superior aspects of the patient's cranium.

The pad of each finger comes into contact with either side of the cranium as follows:

- The little finger, which is nearly parallel to the curved border of the occipital bone, receives the occipital squama.
- The ring finger lies behind the ear at the level of the asterion, with its middle and distal phalanges in contact with the postero-inferior angle of the parietal and mastoid bones respectively.

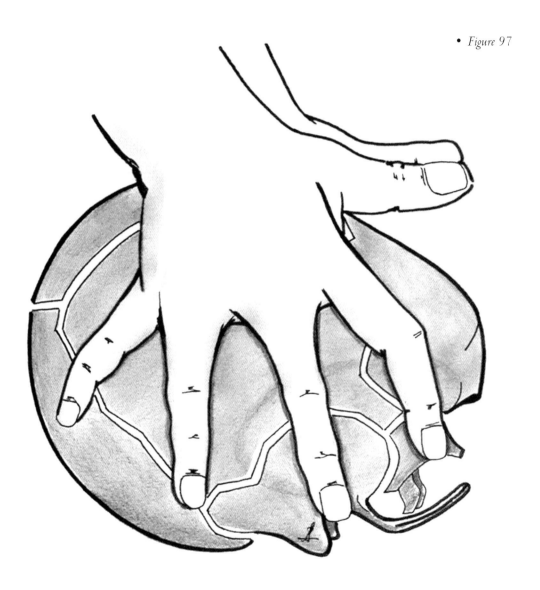

• *Figure 97*

- The middle finger rests in front of the ear, while its middle phalanx (or distal phalanx, depending on the shape of the patient's cranium and of the practitioner's hand) touches the antero-inferior angle of the parietal bone at the level of the pterion.

- The index finger rests on the external surface of the greater wing of the sphenoid.

- One thumb is pressed against the other above the cranium in order to create a fulcrum for the flexor muscles of the fingers.

• *Figure 98*

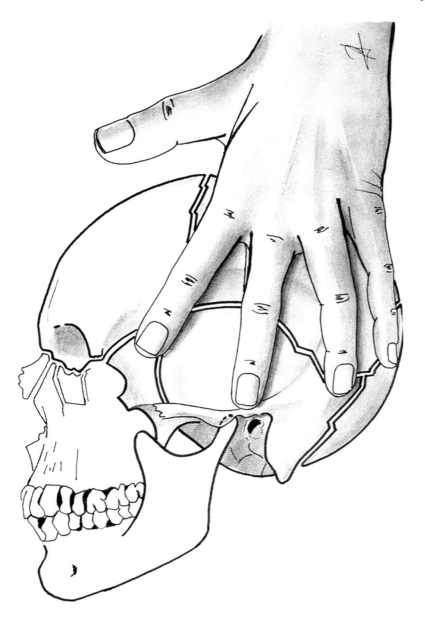

The fronto-occipital approach

This second approach, which is also a classic and often used approach, has the advantage for the therapist that each hand is in a position to receive one of the two bones considered to be the motor components of the cranial system, i.e., the occipital bone in one hand and the sphenoid bone in the other.

The practitioner is still positioned at the head of the patient, but this time to one side or the other. His or her cephalad hand receives the occipital squama, while the other hand cradles the frontal bone and the greater wings of the sphenoid.

The **cephalad hand** (the hand placed posteriorly on the patient's cranium) cups the occipital bone with its fingerpads in contact at the contralateral occipital angle. The angle of the ipsilateral occipital squama lies on the thenar or the hypothenar eminence, or on both of them.

The **caudad hand** (the hand placed anteriorly on the patient's cranium) cups the frontal bone and is in contact with the two external surfaces of the greater wings of the sphenoid. This contact is achieved as follows:

* the pad of the distal phalanx of the index or of the middle finger, or of both these fingers, of the hand on the side opposite the practitioner;
* the pad of the distal phalanx of the thumb on the same side as the practitioner.

• *Figure 99*

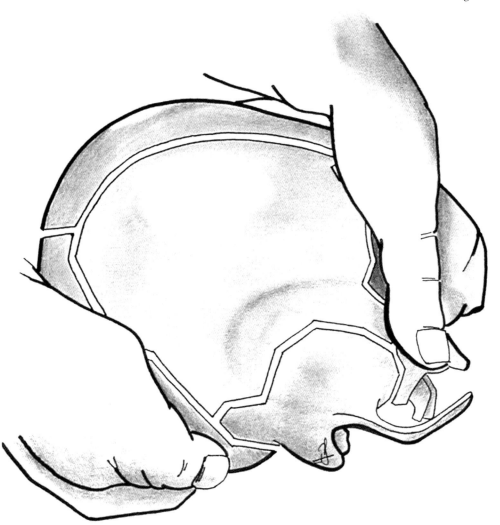

Depending on the width of the first web space (between thumb and index finger), each practitioner will act only on the greater wings of the sphenoid or will also induce motion in the frontal bone.

The diagram on the opposite page and the one on the previous page demonstrate very well the ease with which cranial movements are induced by this approach, and also the loss of ability to feel the specific movements of each of the other bones, in contrast to the preceding approach.

• *Figure 100*

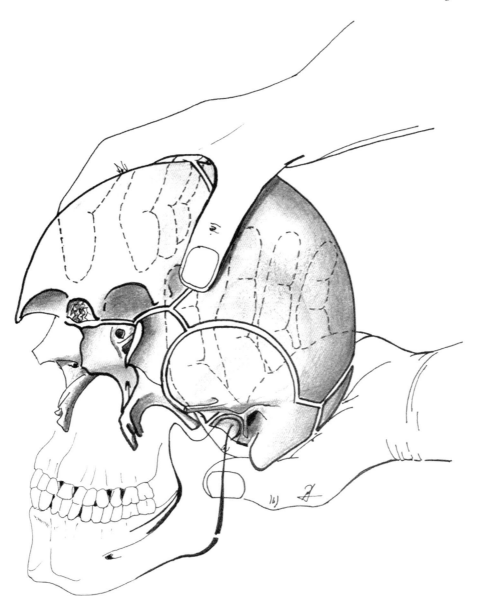

The bimastoid approach

This symmetrical approach has the advantage of using the most important levers of the cranial system (i.e., the mastoid bones), but it also has the drawback that the practitioner is not in direct contact with the motor bones of cranial motion.

We know, however, that using these levers makes this approach more popular for the application of therapeutic techniques, notably those acting on the transverse diameter of the cranium.

The practitioner's hands and interlocked fingers cradle the upper cervical column and the occipital squama. Next, the thumbs, which lie parallel to each other, come to rest along the antero-lateral border of the mastoid processes. The thenar eminences are in contact with the mastoid portions of the temporal bones.

The tip of each thumb lies below the axis of the temporal bone, while its thenar eminence lies above the axis.

The practitioner will then be able to induce any cranial motion starting from the pyramid-shaped petrous portion of the temporal bone, situated like a wedge in the cranial base between the sphenoid anteriorly and the occipital posteriorly.

The tip of each thumb moves posteriorly, medially, and superiorly, inducing flexion, while its thenar eminence moves anteriorly, medially, and superiorly, inducing the opposite movement.

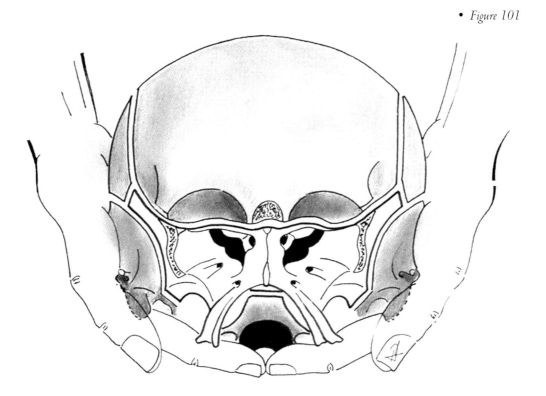

• *Figure 101*

The spheno-mastoid approach

This approach, which is used less often, is a variant of the fronto-occipital approach with the cephalad hand cradling the mastoids instead of the occiput. It is useful not because the movement induced by the practitioner starts from the two motor bones, but because it specifically involves the anterior part of the cranial base (i.e., between the sphenoid and the temporal bones).

The cephalad hand cups the anterior part of the occiput as follows:
- the pad of the thumb touches the ipsilateral mastoid process;
- the pads of the other fingers are pressed together on the contralateral mastoid process.

The caudad hand cups the frontal bone and makes contact with the external surfaces of the greater wings of the sphenoid bone as follows:
- the pad of the distal phalanx of the index finger or of the middle finger, or of both fingers, on the side opposite the practitioner;
- the pad of the distal phalanx of the thumb on the practitioner's side.

• *Figure 102*

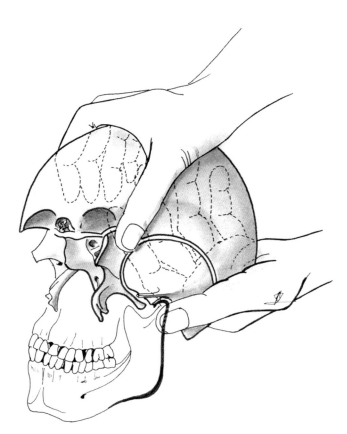

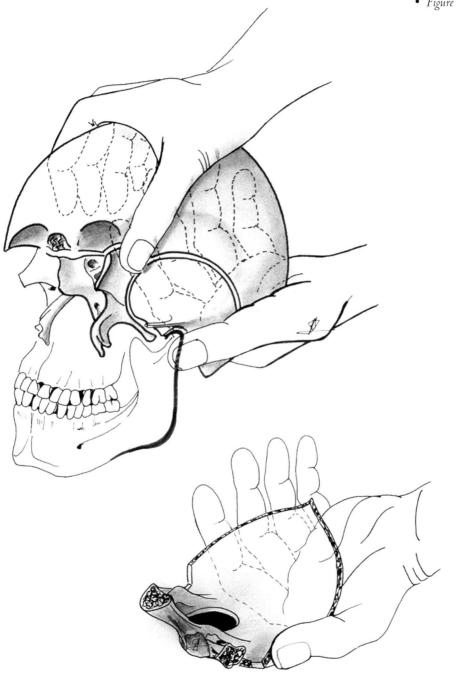

• *Figure 103*

Detection and release of an abnormal bevel

The bevels of the cranial sutures overlap in such a way that, if the therapist pushes them towards each other from the outside, the internal bevel glides on the external bevel over a greater distance than the external bevel, which is limited in its gliding movement over the internal bevel by the epicranial aponeurosis (i.e., the extracranial counterpart to the periosteal layer of the dura mater).

During the release mechanism, the practitioner must first free up the external bevel by pushing it slightly toward the center of the cranium before separating it from the internal bevel, thereby increasing the sutural space.

• *Figure 104*

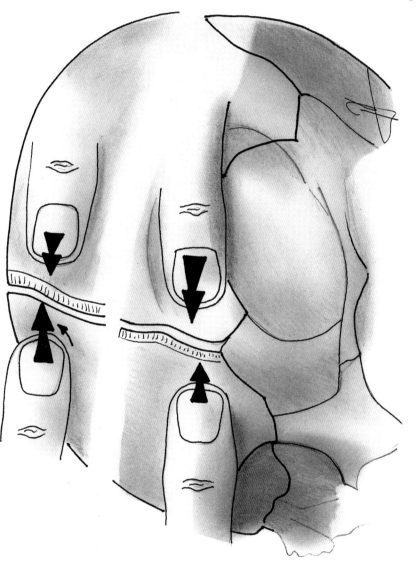

The diagnostic approach

Osteopathic diagnosis

This is carried out in three successive stages:

First, **history-taking**, even if there is no requirement to identify any syndrome, can nonetheless allow the practitioner to make a diagnosis by exclusion. It also allows him or her to use osteopathic reasoning in order to determine the placement of the hands.

Second, **manual examination** allows the practitioner to reveal the physical signs of the lesion.

Finally, two kinds of **tests** are carried out:
- resistance tests confirm the changes in the state of the tissues secondary to the lesion;
- active tests reveal the functional restrictions caused by the lesion.

Manual diagnosis in cranial technique

The vault approach allows the practitioner to make use of the modalities of cranial adaptation (movements of torsion, rotation/lateral flexion, etc.) in order to reveal and confirm which sutures do not open or close normally, and in which quadrant they are located.

In fact, each quadrant contains only one large suture, either in the vault or in the base, with these large sutures linked only by the temporal bone.

Testing the suture suspected of being abnormal then allows the practitioner to identify the lesion precisely and to initiate the appropriate treatment technique.

The protocol thus consists of the successive manual evaluation of the four quadrants united by the temporal bones with its six pivots:

- three at the base;
- three at the vault.

Identification of the four quadrants

On a horizontal section of the cranium, we can imagine two lines intersecting at right angles at a point lying at the center of the cranium (i.e., roughly at the level of the spheno-basilar articulation, deemed to be the motor of cranial motion). As indicated in the diagram on the next page, each quadrant has the following sutural characteristics:

- In the cranial base, each quadrant contains sutures, which become continuous with their contralateral counterparts at the level of the sphenoid:
  - the spheno-frontal sutures in the anterior quadrants;
  - the lambdoid sutures in the posterior quadrants.
- In the cranial vault, there are four sutural articulations (two anterior and two posterior) that join the sagittal suture. These are:
  - the coronal sutures in the anterior quadrants;
  - the lambdoid sutures in the posterior quadrants.

• *Figure 105*

Vault

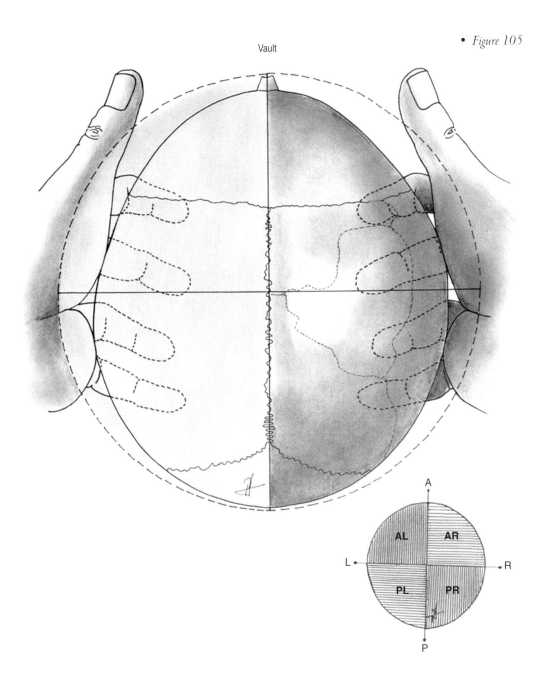

A

AL   AR

L •———   ———• R

PL   PR

P

Manual assessment of the four quadrants

We favor the vault approach, which, as we have already shown, allows us to have contact with each bone and thus to measure the movement of each bone within the general framework of cranial motion.

The two passive hands feel the different components of the spatial motion of each bone, their restrictions, and, in particular, the quality of the end-stage of the movement, which, as we have noted, depends on the state of the connective tissue of the suture.

A lesion in this tissue is followed by a change in its basic properties of flexibility and plasticity, which is caused by an altered blood supply and a loss of its water content.

If the practitioner fails to feel these changes adequately, he or she can impart a slight movement of rebound with the pad of a finger in order to detect the presence or absence of these properties in the connective tissue of the suture being tested.

• *Figure 106*

Base

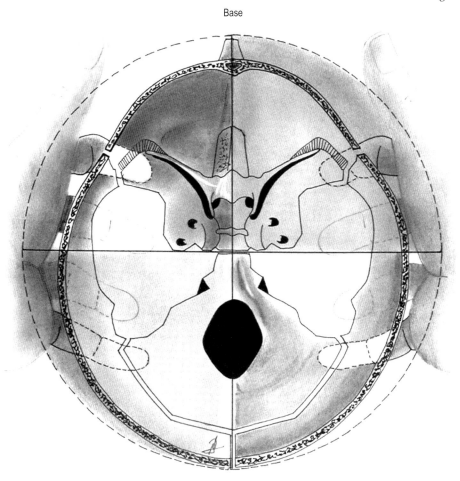

The temporal bone

The temporal bone, which is situated like a wedge at the cranial base, unites the base and the vault as well as the anterior and posterior convexities of the cranium by means of its two orthogonal planes.

Its six pivots, arranged in groups of three along the two orthogonal planes, permit adaptive movements that fine-tune the general motion of the cranium.

Because of this unique function of the temporal bone, we believe that it deserves to be evaluated separately.

• *Figures 107 to 110*

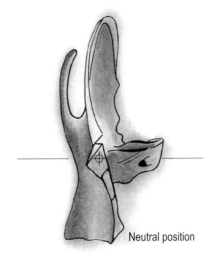

Neutral position

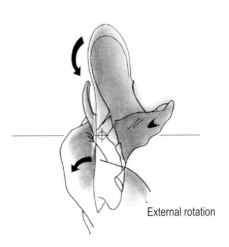

External rotation

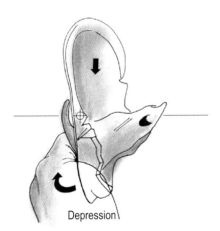

Depression

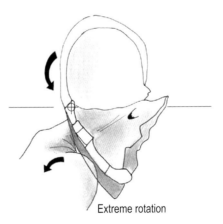

Extreme rotation

Is there a temporal lesion? Where does it lie?

The patient lies supine and relaxed, and the practitioner is positioned at the patient's head. The vault approach consists of the following:

- the little finger below the occiput;
- the index finger along the mastoid process;
- the middle finger in front of the ear;
- the index finger on the external surface of the greater wing of the sphenoid;
- the thumbs touching each other at the sagittal suture and acting as a fulcrum for the diagnostic movements of the fingers that are induced by their flexor muscles.

• *Figure 111*

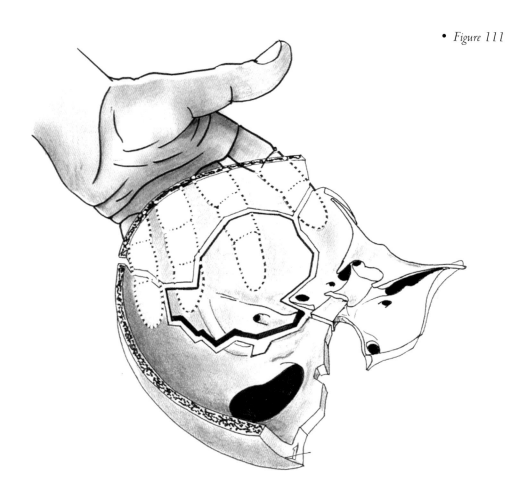

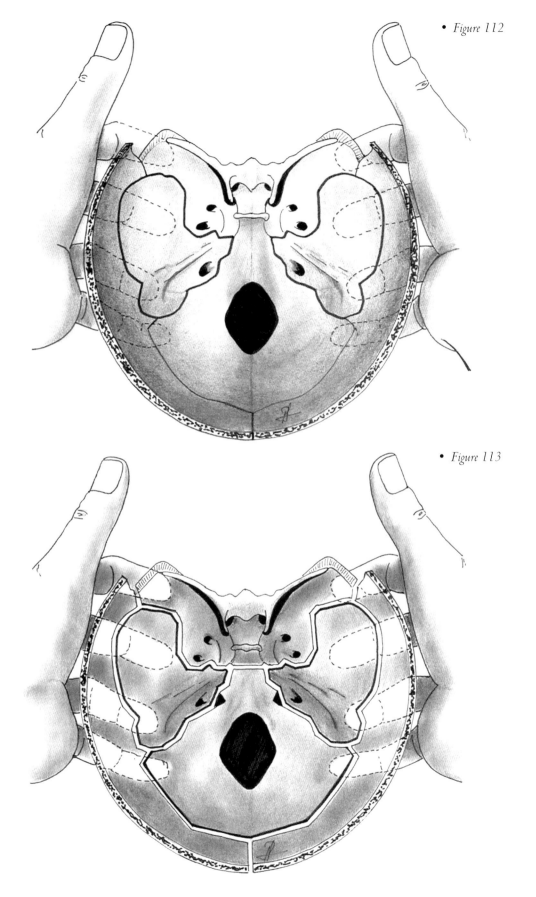

• *Figure 112*

• *Figure 113*

The petro-basilar test

Structural components

This articulation brings the following into contact with each other:

- the superiorly and transversely convex edge of the basilar portion of the occipital bone or the basiocciput;
- the inferiorly and transversely concave edge of the superior portion of the petrous temporal bone.

Movement

This is an external gliding movement of the concave edge of the petrous temporal bone on the convex edge of the basiocciput that causes the cranium to widen transversely during movements of cranial expansion (flexion/external rotation).

The test

From the position described and illustrated in the previous pages, the practitioner evaluates the quality of the final phase of the movement by using the pad of his or her ring finger to impart a "flipper movement" (i.e., a sliding centripetal motion along that transverse axis).

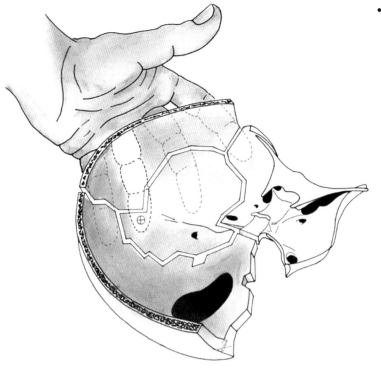

• *Figure 114*

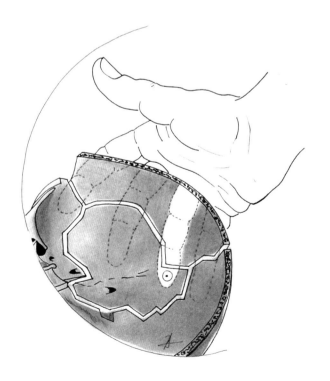

• *Figure 115*

The petro-jugular (petro-occipital) test

Structural components

This synchondrosis brings the following into contact with each other:

- the anterior border of the occipital bone, especially its jugular tubercle, which forms the posterior edge of the jugular foramen;
- the posterior border of the petrous temporal bone, especially its jugular process, which forms the anterior edge of the jugular foramen.

Movement

The jugular foramen is widened. The petrous temporal bone rotates anteriorly on its oblique axis and is slightly depressed while its two borders tend to move apart, thus causing its jugular process to move inferiorly, anteriorly, and slightly medially during the movement of cranial expansion.

The test

Starting from the position we have already described, the practitioner evaluates the quality of the final phase of the movement, as his or her ring finger moves away from the little finger and simultaneously moves inferiorly and slightly medially.

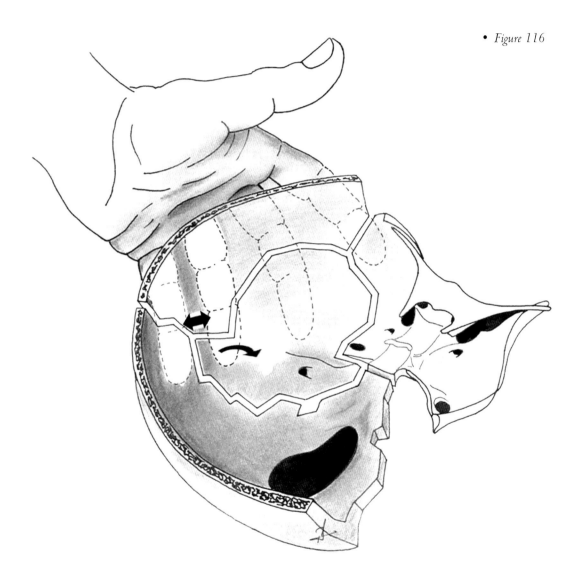

• *Figure 116*

The condylo-squamo-mastoid test

Structural components

This articulation involves the squamous portions of the occipital and temporal bones and brings the following into contact with each other:

- the antero-lateral border of the occipital bone in its squamous region;
- the lanceted posterior border of the petrous portion of the temporal bone.

Movement

This beveled squamous suture is pulled apart, more so in its superior part. Its two constituents (i.e., the occipital and the temporal bones) move posteriorly and inferiorly along non-parallel axes that converge externally and, more importantly, lie in different planes. As a result, these squamous portions of the bones are forced to separate while taking advantage of their plasticity to accommodate the various resulting stresses.

The test

The practitioner evaluates the quality of the final phase of the movement from the starting-point previously defined. His or her ring finger moves away from the little finger while these two fingers are drawn slightly downwards.

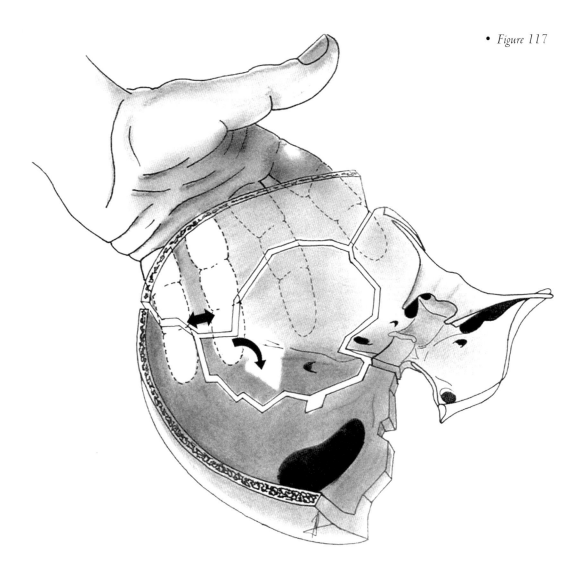

• *Figure 117*

The hinge–mastoid (HM) test

Structural components

This articulation involves the squamous portions of the parietal bone and the temporal squama and brings the following into contact with each other:

- the small bevel lying within the external bevel of the inferior border of the parietal bone;
- the corresponding portion of the superior border of the temporal squama.

We remind the reader that it is this small bevel that allows the temporal bone to shift from external rotation to extreme rotation.

Movement

There is a sliding movement between these two bones, with the temporal squama apparently falling outwards, just like the top of a buckled cartwheel as it sinks into a rut. This release of the HM bevel then allows the temporal bone to enhance its external rotation.

The test

The practitioner evaluates the quality of the final phase of the movement from the starting-point described previously. His or her ring finger barely moves away from the little finger, causing the mastoid to move downwards towards the patient's feet.

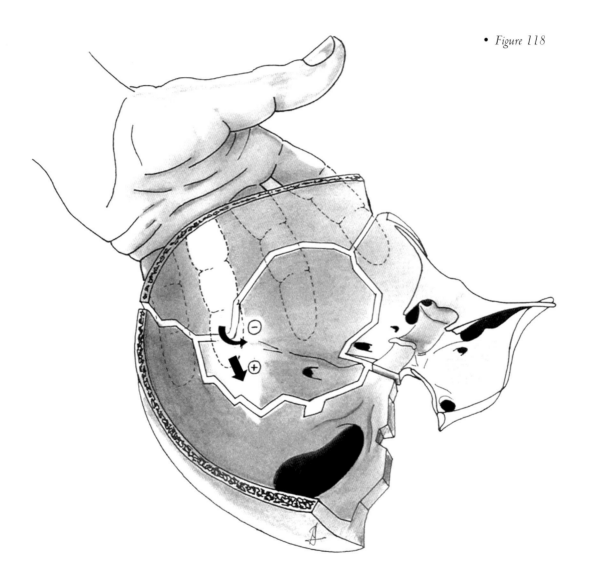

• *Figure 118*

The test for the spheno-squamous pivot

Structural components

This articulation involves the squamous portions of the sphenoid bone and of the temporal squama and brings the following into contact with each other:

- the vertical external and the horizontal internal bevels of the posterior border of the greater wing of the sphenoid, which form a pivot as they change their orientation;
- the corresponding parts of the anterior border of the temporal squama, whose bevels are arranged in the opposite direction.

Movement

The squamous parts of the two bones move apart and rotate anteriorly, slightly laterally, and inferiorly.

The test

The practitioner evaluates the quality of the final phase of the movement from the starting position described previously. His or her index finger moves away from the middle finger, while these two fingers are drawn slightly inferiorly and laterally.

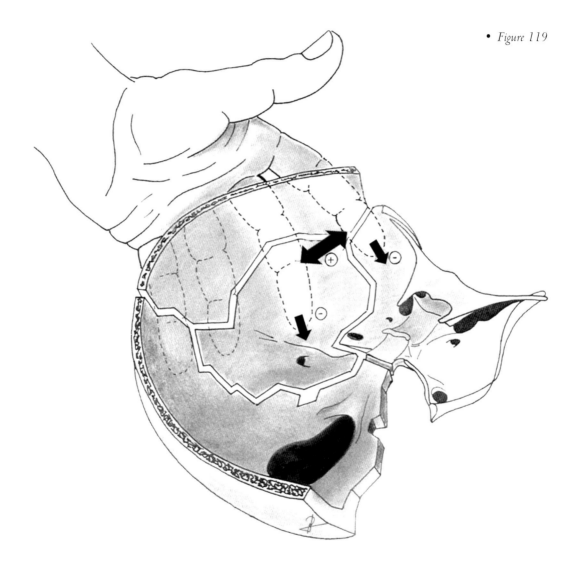

• *Figure 119*

The test for the petro-sphenoid pivot

Structural components

This articulation involves the petro-sphenoid ligament (Grüber's ligament), which is an expansion of the dura mater running from the antero-superior border of the apex of the petrous temporal bone to the posterior clinoid process.

Movement

Circumduction occurs around this ligament (Grüber's ligament), which allows the adaptive movements that must occur at this important anatomical location at the center of the cranial base.

Equally important are the wealth of structures that traverse the cavernous sinus.

The test

The practitioner evaluates the quality of the final phase of the movement from the starting-point described previously. His or her index finger moves slightly away from the middle finger, while the latter finger moves the temporal bone by circumduction, initially inferiorly and then medially, etc.

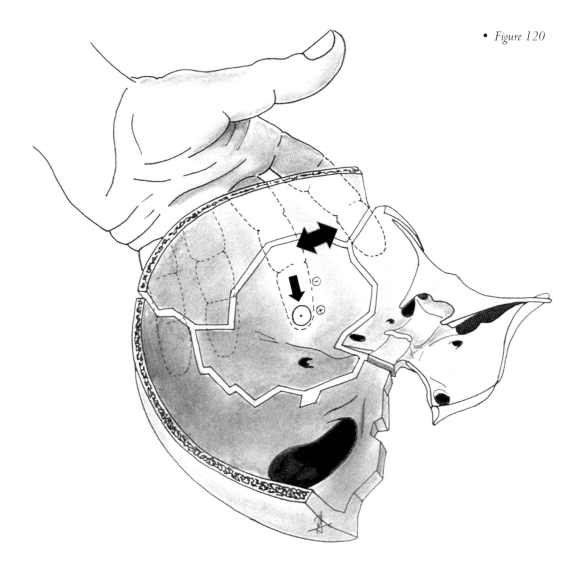

• *Figure 120*

Summary of the tests for the temporal bone pivots

Starting from the "vault approach" position described previously (pp. 134–137), and while maintaining the same contacts continuously, the practitioner will perform the following movements successively and on both sides:

- impart a "flipper movement" with the pad of his or her ring finger for the petro-basilar articulation;

- move his or her ring finger away from the little finger while simultaneously moving it inferiorly and slightly medially for the petro-jugular articulation;

- move his or her ring finger away from the little finger while both are slightly displaced inferiorly for the condylo-squamo-mastoidal pivot;

- move his or her ring finger anteriorly and away from the little finger, and then use it to displace the mastoid downwards for the HM pivot;

- move his or her index finger away from the middle finger while pulling both fingers inferiorly and laterally for the spheno-squamous pivot;

- finally, move his or her index finger away from the middle finger while the latter moves the temporal bone inferiorly and then medially for the spheno-petrous pivot.

• *Figure 121*

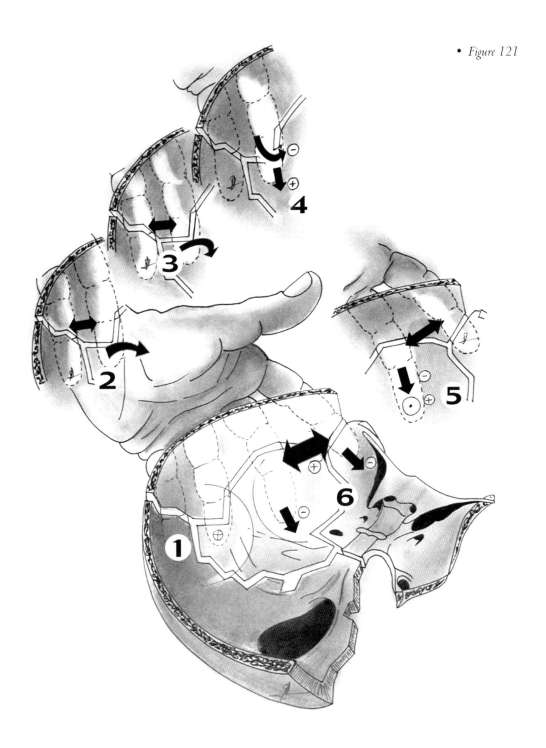

Specific tests for the sphenoid

Intrasphenoidal test (between the body and the greater wings of the sphenoid)

We know that the greater wings of the sphenoid can undergo a very small additional movement with respect to the body at the end of flexion because of a movement of torsion occurring around their sites of attachment. Here, we evaluate this physiological freedom of movement, which is required in times of extra stresses, especially unilateral ones.

The practitioner's position

Level with the patient's head, on one side.

His or her cephalad hand takes hold of the external surface of the two greater wings of the sphenoid in the thumb–index finger pincer, while the pad of the index finger of the caudad hand moves in to touch the hard palate at the cruciform suture.

Movement

The practitioner's hands follow the flexion phase of the midline bones until the end of the movement. While holding the body of the sphenoid in place with the pad of the intraoral index finger, the practitioner then checks whether he or she can still increase the degree of flexion of its greater wings.

• *Figures 122, 123*

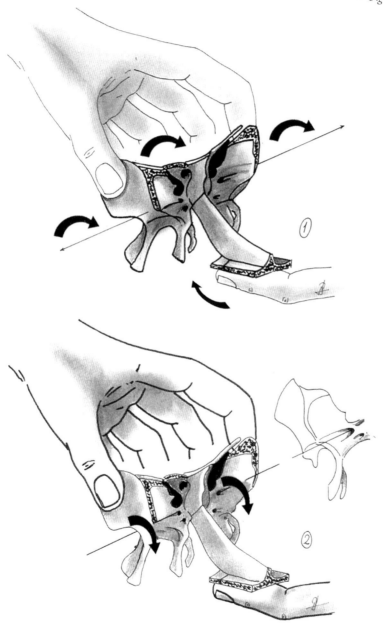

Another intrasphenoidal test

Here, a second type of intrasphenoidal test is carried out by reversing the fixed point. It is particularly useful in cases of entrapment of the trigeminal nerve.

The practitioner's position

Level with the patient's head, to one side.

His or her cephalad hand takes hold of the external surface of the greater wings of the sphenoid in the thumb–index finger pincer, with the pad of the index finger of the caudad hand touching the hard palate at the cruciform suture.

Movement

The practitioner's hands follow the flexion phase of the midline bones until the end of their movement.

While holding the greater wings of the sphenoid in place in the thumb–index pincer, the practitioner checks whether the pad of his or her intraoral finger can still impart a very slight movement to the body of the sphenoid, particularly into extension.

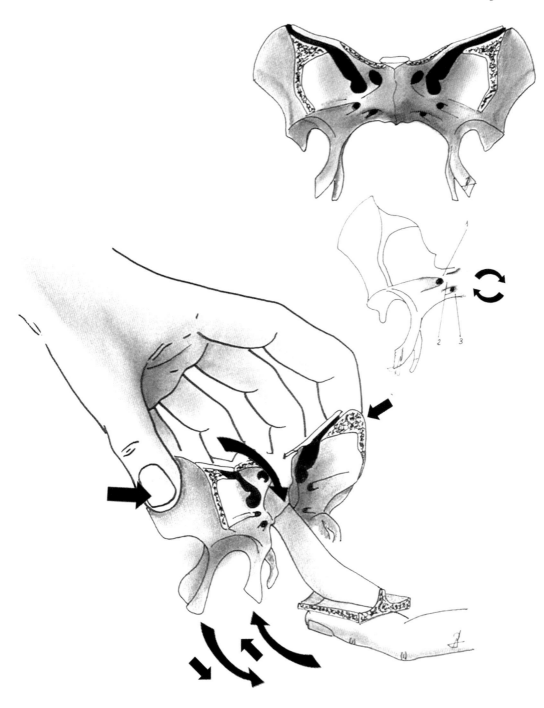

• *Figure 124*

The stylo-hyoid ligament

This ligament acts as a sling for the hyoid bone and stretches from the styloid process of the temporal to the greater horn of the hyoid bone.

The practitioner's position

Level with the patient's head, on one side.

The thumb of his or her cephalad hand lies on the external surface of the contralateral mastoid process, while the thumb–index finger pincer of the caudad hand gently cradles the hyoid bone.

Movement

The thumb of the cephalad hand moves the mastoid process inferiorly, posteriorly, and medially.

The thumb–index finger pincer of the caudad hand gently brings down the hyoid bone toward the sternum, while displacing it to the other side and unwinding it anteriorly.

As soon as tension is felt in the ligament, the practitioner unwinds the ligament around this new axis, which is intended to reveal the most reactive fibers.

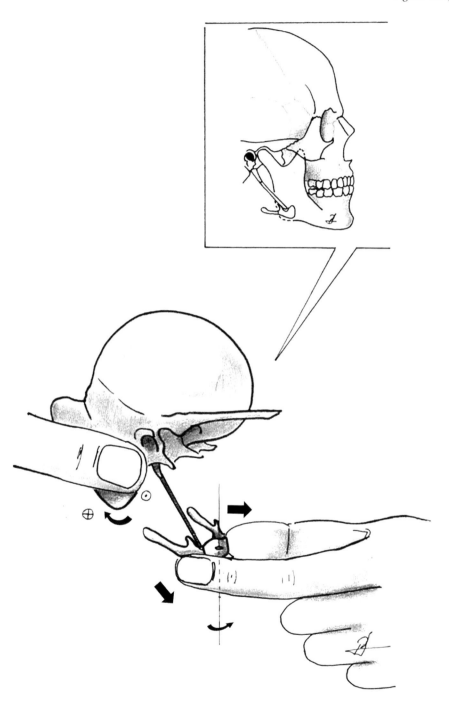

• *Figures 125, 126*

Specific tests for the temporo-mandibular joint

Suspensory ligaments of the mandible

Biomechanically, the temporo-mandibular joints consist of four small joints, two on each side.

On either side there is:

- a temporo-meniscal joint between the temporal bone and the superior aspect of the meniscus;
- a menisco-condylar joint between the inferior aspect of the meniscus and the mandibular condyle.

These joints are attached to a ligamentous system, the importance of which was stressed and illustrated by various studies presented at the 1992 Fourth World Conference of the ICCVT in Washington, DC. We presented our approach to these joints from the cranial osteopathic angle.

The importance of mechanical lesions of the ligaments in the pathology of these joints has since been confirmed. As a corollary, treatment of these ligamentous disturbances can effectively contribute to the management of diseases of these joints.

We will now present the tests that allow us to identify and to differentiate among these diseases.

The stylo-mandibular (temporo-mandibular) ligament

This fibrous band runs from the styloid process of the temporal bone to the inferior angle of the mandible. Its lower attachment acts as the center of rotation for the mandible during the first phase of opening the mouth, when the meniscus is bent superiorly and anteriorly under the pressure exerted by the condyle.

The practitioner's position

At the patient's head, to one side.

The thumb of the practitioner's cephalad hand is placed on the ipsilateral mastoid process, while the caudad hand grasps the contralateral mandible between the thumb, which lies on the postero-medial part of the body of the mandible, and the index and middle fingers, which lie externally behind and below the gonion respectively.

Movement

The thumb of the practitioner's cephalad hand moves the mastoid process inferiorly, posteriorly, and medially. The other hand moves the mandible, first anteriorly (the first phase of opening the patient's mouth) and then inferiorly and anteriorly while tilting it very slightly to the other side.

As soon as tension is felt in the ligaments, the practitioner unwinds the ligament around this new axis in order to identify its most reactive fibers.

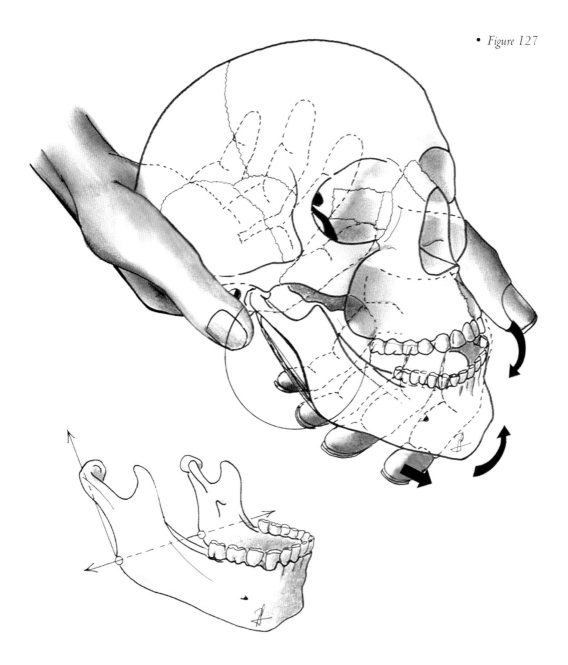

• *Figure 127*

The spheno-mandibular ligament

This fibrous band stretches from the spine of the sphenoid to the lingula of the mandible. Its lower attachment acts as a center of rotation for the mandible during the second phase of opening the mouth (the mouth wide open).

The practitioner's position

At the head of the patient, to one side.

The practitioner's cephalad hand grips the greater wings of the sphenoid in the thumb–index finger pincer, while the caudad hand grips the contralateral mandible between the thumb, which lies on the postero-medial part of the body of the mandible, and the index and middle fingers, which lie externally behind and below the gonion respectively.

Movement

The practitioner's cephalad hand follows the sphenoid into flexion, and the caudad hand first moves the mandible in such a way as to open the mouth fully and then inferiorly and posteriorly while tilting it very slightly to one side.

As soon as tension is felt in the ligaments, the practitioner unwinds the ligament around this new axis in order to identify its most reactive fibers.

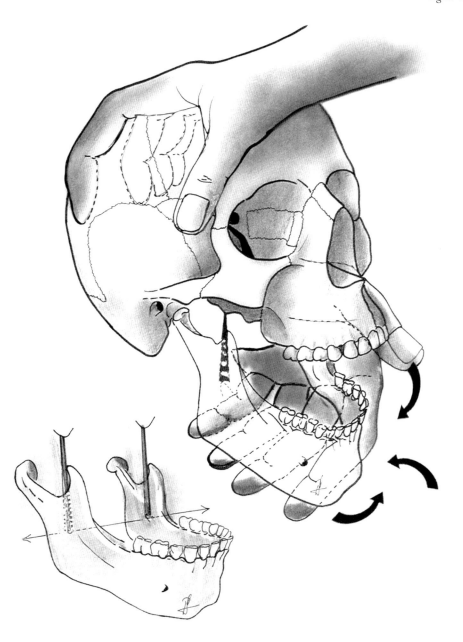

• *Figure 128*

The lateral collateral ligament

This strong triangular ligament extends from the articular tubercle at the root of the zygomatic process of the temporal bone to the postero-lateral surface of the neck of the mandibular condyle and to the meniscus.

The practitioner's position

The practitioner stands at the head of the patient, whose face is turned away, and places the pad of the thumb of his or her cephalad hand behind the condyle in the tiny fossa formed as the patient half opens his or her mouth. The pad of the thumb of the practitioner's caudad hand rests against and behind the other thumb.

Movement

The posterior thumb pushes on the other thumb, pulling the mandibular condyle anteriorly toward the orbit until tension is felt in the ligaments. The quality of this tension in terms of the ligament's elasticity and plasticity is a reflection of its condition.

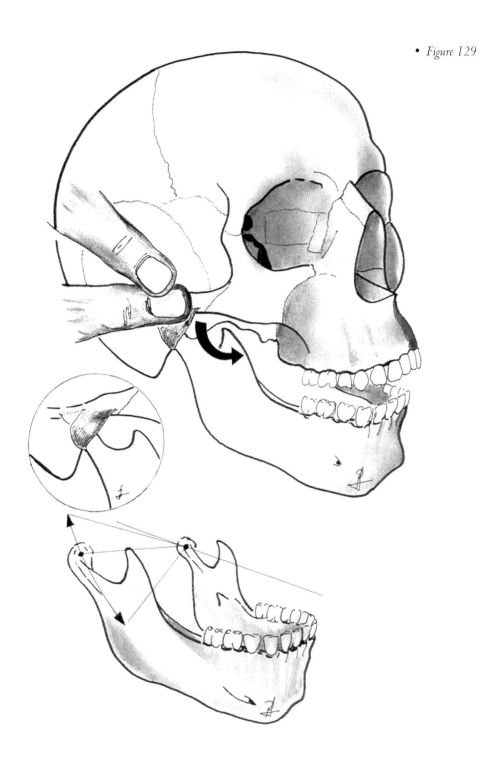

• *Figure 129*

Test for the meniscus of the temporo-mandibular joint

This test allows us to assess to what degree the meniscus has preserved its ability to adapt to the various physiological stresses.

The practitioner's position

At the patient's head, with the patient's face turned toward the practitioner. This test is carried out on the contralateral joint.

The practitioner's cephalad hand controls the temporal bone with the index finger lying anterior and the middle finger posterior to the mastoid, while the thumb is placed on the patient's cheek over the place corresponding to the meniscus (i.e., between the mandibular fossa of the temporal bone and the mandibular condyle).

The caudad hand grasps the mandible between the thumb placed on the postero-medial part of the body of the mandible and the index and middle fingers placed on the outside of the mandible behind and below the gonion respectively.

Assessment

The temporal bone is pulled into external rotation during the expansion phase of the cranial system, while the hand on the mandible tests the following movements in succession: anterior translation, rotation of the condyle on its transverse axis, adduction–abduction, vertical rotation, lateral displacement, and lateral inclination.

Specific tests for the ocular muscles

Tests for the different ocular muscles

Although the extrinsic eye muscles are all inserted into the sclera, their insertions are nonetheless quite distinct from one another. All these muscles, except for the inferior oblique, have a common tendinous origin on the internal surface of the superior orbital fissure of the sphenoid bone (the tendon of Zinn).

Purpose

These techniques will allow the practitioner to evaluate the tension in the various extrinsic muscles of each eye and to detect any possible imbalance.

Position of the patient and of the practitioner

The patient lies supine in a comfortable and relaxed position, with eyes closed.

The practitioner is to one side of the patient's head.

Contact points

The practitioner's cephalad hand grasps the greater wings of the sphenoid in the thumb–index finger pincer.

The caudad hand is in gentle contact with the eyeball via three splayed out fingers (thumb, index, and middle fingers).

Tests for the rectus muscles of the eye

These muscles run from the common tendinous ring (the tendon of Zinn) on the sphenoid bone to the following:

- the lateral surface of the sclera for the lateral rectus;
- the inferior surface of the sclera for the inferior rectus;
- the medial surface of the sclera for the medial rectus;
- the superior surface of the sclera for the superior rectus.

Strict attention must be paid to the exact positions of the patient and practitioner, as described in the preceding pages, and the evaluation procedure is carried out in the following way.

The practitioner's cephalad hand moves the patient's sphenoid bone into flexion, while the caudad hand gently rotates the eyeball in a direction that is opposite to the insertion site of the muscle under scrutiny, as follows:

- laterally for the medial rectus;
- medially for the lateral rectus;
- inferiorly for the superior rectus;
- superiorly for the inferior rectus.

As soon as the practitioner feels any tension, he or she asks the patient to look in the direction of the muscle under scrutiny (e.g., medially for the medial rectus) with eyes closed. The practitioner can then easily sense whether the tension is normal or not.

• *Figure 130*

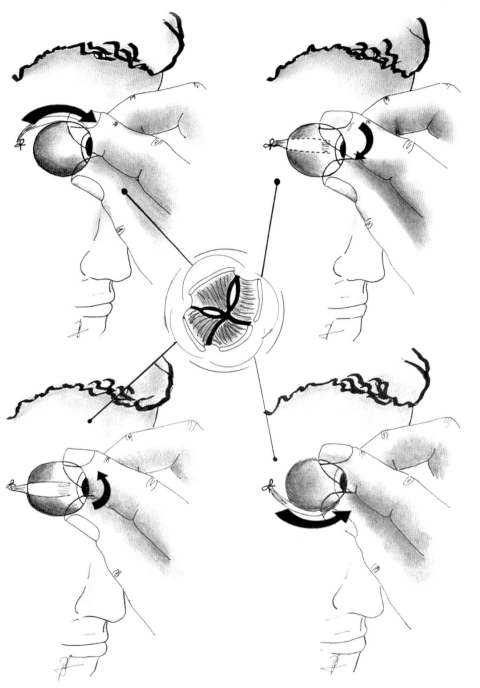

Test for the superior oblique muscle of the eye

This muscle runs from the lesser wing of the sphenoid above the optic foramen to the supero-lateral surface of the eyeball.

It moves the cornea laterally and inferiorly.

It is the most important muscle for reading.

Strict attention must be paid to the exact positions of the patient and practitioner, as described previously (p. 187), and the evaluation procedure is carried out as follows. The practitioner's cephalad hand moves the patient's sphenoid bone into flexion, while the caudad hand gently rotates the eyeball in the direction opposite to the insertion site of the superior oblique muscle (i.e., inferiorly and anteriorly).

As soon as the practitioner feels any tension, he or she asks the patient, whose eyes are still closed, to look downwards and inwards and then upwards and inwards. The practitioner can then easily sense whether or not the tension is normal.

• *Figure 131*

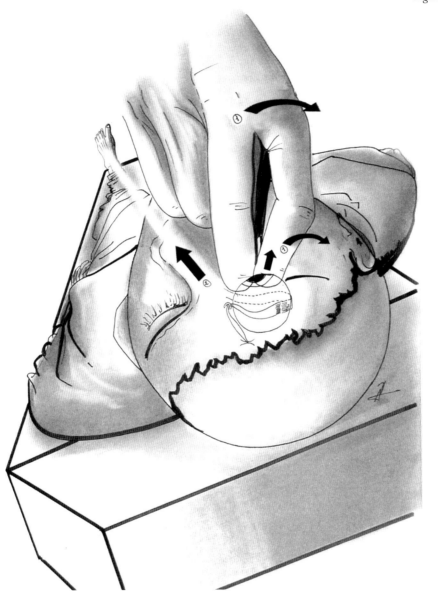

Test for the inferior oblique muscle of the eye

This muscle runs from the osseous border of the upper opening of the naso-lacrimal canal to the infero-lateral part of the posterior aspect of the eyeball.

It moves the cornea laterally and superiorly.

Strict attention must be paid to the positions of both patient and practitioner, as described previously (p. 187), and the evaluation procedure is carried out as follows.

The practitioner's caudad hand moves the patient's maxilla into external rotation, while the cephalad hand gently rotates the eyeball in the direction opposite to the insertion site of the inferior oblique (i.e., inferiorly and medially).

As soon as the practitioner feels any tension, he or she asks the patient, whose eyes are still closed, to look upwards and outwards. The practitioner can then easily sense whether the tension is normal or not.

• *Figure 132*

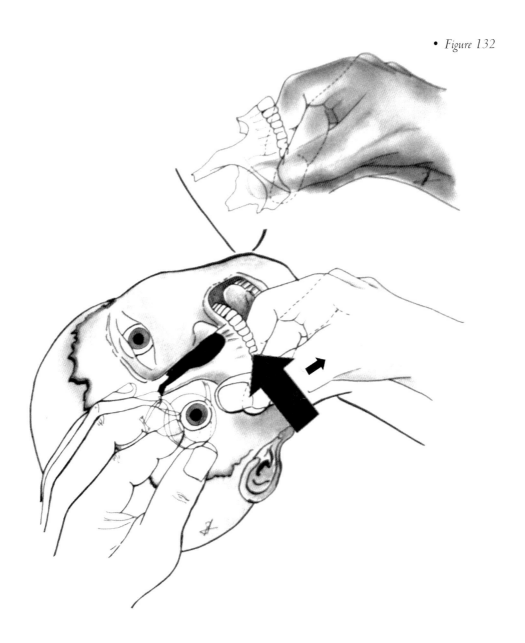